Contents

Acknowledgements

I must say thankyou to all those midwives who have given me, so freely over the years, their support and advice and to the women who have given me the privilege of being at the birth of their children. I'd also like to thank Catherine, Emma (and Henry, of course) at Books for Midwives Press for their patient understanding! As before, my deepest love and thanks must go to those closest to me – my parents, Tom and Mary Russell, and my beloved husband Pete, without whose encouragement, love and support, none of the things I've achieved in my life would ever have happened.

Thanks to Michael Melotte for his work on the insurance chapter and to Frances Webb who wrote the chapter on marketing.

Introduction

When I wrote the first edition of *The Independent Midwife*, I thought the readership would be somewhat specialized. I (and Books for Midwives Press, I suspect) were slightly stunned when it sold so well – so much so that copies have been purloined from libraries. Always a sign, I have been told, of a popular book!

Under the circumstances, therefore, it seemed sensible to do a new edition. However, there have been a few major events since then. The vexed question of professional indemnity insurance remains unsolved at the time of writing, as do issues of midwife-led care, one-to-one provision, individualized care, underfunding of the NHS and so on. The book, therefore, is still aimed at those of you who feel the need to find out how to take that huge step out of the mainstream and what it means to 'go independent'.

As I said last time, welcome to the world of autonomous practice.

Lesley Hobbs
July 1997

CHAPTER ONE

Setting the Scene

Since time began, midwives have been supporting pregnant and labouring women, assisting them to deliver their babies, and, probably, making the tea afterwards. The midwife has been the Wise Woman, the fount of female knowledge, and on occasion, reviled for being just that. If you look back to relatively recent history, you will see many of the wise women perceived as witches – and getting burned at the stake as a consequence.

Now the midwifery profession stands on the brink, at risk this time, not of being burnt, but of being set aside in favour of technology. Technology, in its place, is not a bad thing, but do not be fooled – it in no way replaces the skills and the art of a midwife.

'Midwife' means 'with woman' (mid-wif). It is precisely that aspect which has brought many of us to the midwifery profession. Our role is to advise, assist, listen to, and meet the needs of the women in our care. We are their attendants; as such, we should ensure that the care we give is fitted to that woman's needs. She should not have to fit herself into an institutional framework that sees her as a passive recipient of care, rather than an active participant in it.

We have found our traditional role being gradually eroded. Our specialized training is being subsumed into the higher education model, and our disciplinary procedures taken over by a system comprising mostly nurses. Now, before it is too late, we feel it is time that midwives re-established the basic role of the midwife. We are autonomous practitioners, and the prime advocates for the childbearing woman.

Just how wide ranging is our professional responsibility? The definition of a midwife, amended by the International Confederation of Midwives Council in 1990, and ratified by the International Federation of Gynaecologists and Obstetricians in 1991 and the World Health Organization in 1992, is as follows:

'A midwife is a person who, having been regularly admitted to a midwifery educational programme, duly recognized in the country in which it is located, has successfully completed the prescribed course of studies in midwifery and has acquired the requisite qualifications to be registered and/or legally licensed to practise midwifery.

She must be able to give the necessary supervision, care and advice to women during pregnancy, labour and the postpartum period, to conduct deliveries on her own responsibility and to care for the newborn and the infant. This care includes preventative measures, the detection of abnormal conditions in mother and child, the procurement of medical assistance and the execution of emergency measures in the absence of medical help. She has an important task in health counselling and education, not only for the women, but also within the family and community. The work should involve antenatal education and preparation for parenthood, and extends to certain areas of gynaecology, family planning and child care. She may practise in hospitals, clinics, health units, domiciliary conditions or in any other service.' (World Health Organization, 1992)

How many midwives can put their hands on their hearts and say that they truly practise to the full extent of the role? Most midwives are hedged about with hospital policies. Many of these policies have no basis in research, and some may even be harmful to women subjected to them. As an example, one only has to consider the folly of depriving a woman of food and nourishing fluids when she is in labour, and working harder than at any other time in her life (Enkin, Keirse and Chalmers, 1995).

Having said all that, however, it is a very safe feeling to work within the confines of a large institution. The concept of autonomous practice does not figure largely within the framework of hospital policy. Many midwives feel much more comfortable working in a place where medical back-up is a constant presence. Some midwives are not even aware of independent midwifery, and seem to think that hospital based practice is the only option. In reality, a midwife can actually start practising independently as soon as she qualifies, although very few do that. Most practice within the NHS for a while after registering.

So, why go it alone? Why leave the warm security of the institution for the uncertainties of independent practice? Those currently practising independently have many reasons, but the prime reason for all seems to be that they are unable to practise fully as a midwife within the confines of current hospital systems. Often it appears that women's needs come second to the needs of the institution. Staffing requirements dictate that women may have to wait for hours in antenatal clinics; may have to share their midwife on labour ward with one, two or even three other women; and that their time on the postnatal ward is characterized by heat, noise, conflicting advice and meals at all the wrong times! Even community midwives are bound by policies on who they may or may not accept for a homebirth – not realizing, or choosing to mislead women about, the fact that it is the woman's right to choose where and how she has her baby. As professionals, we can only advise. We should not compel, or coerce, or blackmail women into doing as we think best. There is evidence, however, that these tactics are being used all too often.

There are uncertainties in independent practice, as in any self-employed occupation. Aspects of these will be discussed in detail in later chapters. It is important for any would-be independent practitioner to lay her plans meticulously, and well in advance. The positive side of independent practice is based upon the knowledge that the service provided at least gives women the opportunity to make their own decisions, in possession of the information necessary to make those decisions.

Independents are often perceived as mavericks; natural rebels against authority, iconoclasts, boat rockers. Well, yes, to an extent that may be so. However, without challenge, there is no change; without grit, there is no pearl; without independents, there would be nothing for the hospital-based system to measure itself against. If the system feels itself threatened, then there must be something in the system that is capable of being threatened. That something is, I believe, contained in the way in which institutions treat pregnant women, regarding them, in general, as unfit vessels for the task of childbearing. This attitude is already the subject of several books, so there is nothing to be gained by going into detail here. Suffice it to say, that any woman who chooses to go outside the system to find a midwife wants to know that her needs and wishes will be respected, and that her decisions will be regarded as having been made by a proper grown-up person.

Independent midwives do not, however, do it alone. Although some midwives do practise single-handed, the majority work in partnerships, or practices of three or more. This enables midwives to have time off, and to remind themselves of what their own family looks like, and where they live. These little points tend to get forgotten when practices get really busy.

There is a network of support already in existence, covering all facets of working and practice, and in addition, all independent midwives should make a point of getting to know all their local pressure groups (see Appendix 7). Not only will these groups help by spreading the word about independents and their practices, but also act as an information resource. Ignore them at your peril.

As far as practical help goes, make use of the professional organizations. The Independent Midwives Association (IMA) provides information, workshops, meetings and encouragement. They may also know of other independents in your area, who can help you in starting your practice and give you useful local information. Independents tend to rely on each other a lot for support, advice and, importantly, companionship. Professional isolation can be a most demoralizing experience. Often independents in one area will get together on a regular basis just to talk, in addition to the regular meetings held by the association. The IMA produces a register of independent midwives which is updated twice a year. This register is sent to anyone wanting information on independent midwives, and is a marvellous source of publicity. Payment of a small fee will give you access to all the benefits of the association, and put your name in the register.

The Royal College of Midwives is the professional body for all practising midwives, and has the expertise necessary for advising on any issues regarding the practice or profession of midwifery. They do not provide indemnity insurance for independents (see Chapter 2 – Legal Issues) but can be contacted for other types of specialist insurance. They can also help you to avoid mistakes by giving opinions on such matters as notes, or advertising, for example, before you commit yourself to print.

Summary

Finally, don't rush it. Once you have made the decision to start in independent practice, it can be very tempting to just go for it. Hold on to the following thoughts:

1. You need to support yourself unless you have inherited a sizeable fortune, or have a partner who makes enough to support you both. Don't give up the day job until you have clients booked.

2. Buy yourself only the basic minimum of equipment you need to start (see list in Chapter 3). That way, if you don't enjoy working independently you haven't wasted your money.

3. Talk to other independent practitioners, spend some time with them if you can, and try to attend a workshop or study day.

4. Read this book from cover to cover.

Then go for it.

CHAPTER TWO

Legal Issues

The legal framework surrounding the practice of midwifery is based upon the Nurses, Midwives and Health Visitors Act 1992. This Act superseded the 1979 Act, following the Government's review (by Peat Marwick McClintok) of the Statutory Body system in 1989. At the time of writing, the bodies relevant to midwifery are the National Boards for England, Scotland, Wales and Northern Ireland (the NBs) and the United Kingdom Central Council for Nursing, Midwifery and Health Visiting (UKCC).

Procedural committees
UKCC complaints procedure
Until recently, it has been the responsibility of the relevant National Board to screen, and investigate initially, complaints of alleged professional misconduct. Since April 1st 1993, this system has changed. From that date, all allegations of professional misconduct will go directly to the new Preliminary Proceedings Committee at the UKCC. This committee functions in a similar way to the former Investigating committee, has the same responsibilities, and can take the same decisions:

1.   To take no further action.
2.   To refer on to the Professional Conduct Committee, with a view to removal from the register on the grounds of professional misconduct.
3.   To refer on to the Health Committee with a view to removal/ suspension from the register on the grounds of ill-health.

There is one major difference however, and that is that the new committees will have the option on a fourth decision. Since April 1st, they have been able to administer a caution to the practitioner. This will remain on the practitioner's records at the UKCC (and nowhere else) for a period of five years. *The caution can only be administered if the midwife admits the facts, and the consequent misconduct. In the case of the preliminary proceedings committee, even if the midwife does admit the facts, she may still be referred on, if the committee feels this to be the right course of action, rather than issuing a caution.*

Referral to either of the two committees does not necessarily mean being removed from the register. The Health Committee can, if it seems appropriate, issue a simple suspension, which means that the midwife will not be returned to the register until her health is satisfactory. The Professional Conduct Committee has to consider whether misconduct has been proven to its satisfaction, and if it has, to consider what action to take. There are four options:

1.   To take no action.
2.   To administer a caution (see above).
3.   To postpone judgement – this means that the practitioner will be set goals which must be achieved by the time the committee meets again to consider the case. The judgement will be given at this follow-up session.
4.   To remove the practitioner from the register.

With regard to suspension from practice, see Chapter 6 'Supervision'.

Every midwife should be so familiar with the form and content of the Midwives Rules and Code of Practice that she can quote the appropriate section if required. This is especially true of independent practitioners. The information contained in these documents is intended to ensure safe practice, and to protect the public. Read, remember and inwardly digest. Never make assumptions on matters concerning the Rules or the Code of Practice. Always check, if you are unclear on any issue, with the relevant National Board, the Royal College of Midwives or directly with the UKCC.

There are a series of documents relating to practice, and issued by the UKCC. These include guidance on Advertising, Confidentiality and the Code of Professional Conduct for the Nurse, Midwife and Health Visitor. You will need all these, and should obtain them from the UKCC at the address at the end of the book in Appendix 7.

Red hot record keeping

The next issue of importance to the independent practitioner is the thorny question of record keeping. When working in the hospital based system, records tend to be brief. As an independent, you need to be sure that your records are as listed below.

Contemporaneous

They must be kept as contemporaneously as possible. Do your best to write them as you go along. It doesn't matter if they get liquor, meconium or coffee on them as long as they are still legible, you can always copy them out again. Stains are a hazard of the business. Don't be tempted to leave it and write them up afterwards. You'll leave out something important, and it will come back and haunt you ten years later.

Approval of format

They must be in a form approved by the Local Supervising Authority. This means that if you devise your own records (as most do), then they must be approved by your Supervisor. It is a good idea to view designing your records as part of an evolutionary process – you'll frequently think of a better way of doing one part or the other. You may be offered hospital notes to use, but this is not always a good idea. For one thing, if they are marked with the name of the hospital, it can be difficult to establish ownership, and for another they may not be in a format which is best for you and your clients.

All your records should be clear, unambiguous, easy to read and written in ink which is not likely to fade over the twenty five years you're required to keep them. The more detail you put in the better. Each entry must be accurate in date and time, and clearly signed. Any alterations must be made by crossing out with a single line, and the additional entry dated, timed and signed. You should make sure that you don't include 'abbreviations, meaningless phrases and offensive subjective statements unrelated to the patient's care and associated observations' (as if you would!). For further detail on records and record keeping, read the UKCC's paper on 'Standards for records and record keeping', published by the Council in April 1993 (see Appendix 3 for examples of notes format).

Storage

You must keep them in a safe place, away from curious eyes. If you are not able to do this, or when you stop practising as an independent, you should arrange for the Health Authority to take them into care. Details of this transfer should be kept by both parties. It's a good idea to keep them in the back of a locked filing cabinet, or in a fireproof box. If anything happens to your notes, such as a house fire, then you will really be in difficulties. Some midwives make copies of their notes and ask their Supervisors to look after them in the medical records department. This is much the same as making backups on a computer. Speaking of which, if you decide to keep notes on disk, you may have to register yourself under the Data Protection Act. This may also apply to databases, and audits of records. Contact the Data Protection Agency for detailed information, as the need for registration may vary according to the nature of the data on disk.

Sharing input

It is an indication of the partnership between the independent and her client that the client also has a full copy of the notes. These can be used in a similar way to co-op cards if a GP is sharing care, or if a referral to a medical practitioner is indicated. These notes can be used as a diary of the pregnancy with the woman contributing to the entries, or she could be given a photocopy at the end. Women love to have these notes, looking on them largely as a memento of the big event.

You may also like to keep your old diaries with the notes, as these also provide a record of visits. Many midwives find it useful to have a page in the notes where communications from colleagues, such as Supervisors and GPs can be recorded.

Formal records of visits made are contained in the Registers of Cases I and II. The first register should contain details of all visits made to clients, and the second detailed reports on all deliveries. It may be useful for you to include extra details in the second register, such as blood loss, for example. There is plenty of space in each column for additional information – you don't have to stick to the basics. These extra details will be useful to you when you come to the annual audit of your practice. You can obtain these books from the Canterbury Press (Norwich), Hymns Ancient and Modern, St Mary's work, St Mary's Plain, Norwich, Norfolk, NR3 3BH, Tel: 01603 616563. They cost £7.11 (including postage) for the pair.

Continuing education

PREP

All midwives have an obligation to keep up to date with their practice, and the UKCC Post Registration Education and Practice (PREP) regulations are intended to formalize a record of your experiences and achievements, as well as enabling all practitioners to have access to further education, training and return to work schemes.

Refresher courses

If you intend practising for more than three years after qualifying, the issue of refresher courses will become relevant. The Rules state that every midwife,

> 'who gives notice of intention to practice under Rule 36 shall within 12 months of notifying such intention complete a course of instruction or provide evidence of appropriate professional education approved by a Board for the purpose of this Rule'.

This does not apply to:

1. Midwives who qualified, or who have attended a refresher course less than three years ago; or
2. Midwives who, because they have not practised as a midwife for the equivalent of 12 working weeks during the preceding five years, need to attend a four week course at an approved training institution.

Study days

There are several options on refresher courses, which comes as a great relief to midwives who did not want, or could not afford, to spend a week on a study course. You can now build up refresher days over the three years, at specific events which interest you. All you have to make sure is that the study day you are attending has NB approval. You will need five of these days. They also cost money in small chunks (£30–45) rather than the large amount (£250–350) which the week long courses cost.

NB courses

You may also use certain National Board courses as refresher course substitutes. Please note that the National Board course numbers are the same in England, Scotland, Wales and Northern Ireland. All the following are examples of courses which can be used.

*   NB 405 Special and Intensive Nursing Care of the Newborn. 24 weeks.
*   870 An Introduction to the Understanding and Application of Research. 40 days.
*   901 Family Planning. 10 days theory. 12 clinical sessions.
*   934 Care and Management of Persons with Acquired Immune Deficiency Syndrome (AIDS) and Human Immuno-deficiency Virus (HIV) – related conditions. Minimum 10 days.
*   985 Principles of Psychosexual Counselling. 20–30 days.
*   997 Teaching and Assessing in Clinical Practice. 15 days minimum.
*   A08 Advanced Family Planning. Minimum 40 days.

Alternatives to refresher courses

You may, if you wish, design your own refresher course. This may be a period of two weeks planned practical experience. You need to discuss, with your Supervisor and a midwife teacher, what your learning needs are, how the learning outcomes can be identified at the end of your course and the form and nature of the theoretical basis for your course. Some midwives like the opportunity to refurbish their skills in a hospital setting.

This has the added advantage (at the moment) of not costing anything. The course plan will then be submitted, by the Supervisor, to the relevant NB for formal approval.

Other refresher opportunities include undertaking courses designed to lead to a further professional qualification or which otherwise enhance your practice. These include the Diploma in Professional Studies (Midwifery), formerly the Advanced Diploma in Midwifery, and an education course enabling you to become a teacher of midwives. It is useful to note that if you do these courses by the distance learning route, the first module counts as a refresher course in itself. If you take a degree course, then this can be counted as a refresher provided that:

1.   The course will enhance your practice as a midwife, and
2.   That the dissertation is on an aspect of midwifery.

Finally, you may be involved with a substantial research project, or even writing a book, which will enhance your practice. You can ask your Supervisor to submit this for approval as a refresher course. Do bear in mind that either Supervisor or the NB may not accept it in lieu of a more conventional refresher course, but it's always worth trying.

In the normal way, all refresher courses which do not come under the heading of NB approved study days or refresher courses will be notified to the relevant NB, by your Supervisor, for the Board's approval. If you are at university or college full-time, and therefore do not have a current Supervisor, you can submit your plan to the NB yourself. However, it helps to ring them first and have a chat about it before you submit it, as this will give you any necessary guidance on what, exactly, is likely to be useful.

Funding

As an independent, you will, unfortunately, have to fund this yourself (but it is tax deductible), unless you can find another source of funding, such as a charitable sponsor. There is no point in looking to either the Department of Trade and Industry or the Training and Enterprise Council for help. The only government funding available for this sort of thing is in the form of a loan. This is interest free, but must be repaid three months after the course is completed – ask the Department of Employment for details.

In order to find out what courses are available, you could read the lists in publications such as the MIDIRS digest, and then apply, but courses, especially popular ones, do get booked up very early. It is perhaps better to contact the National Board in advance and ask the appropriate education officer what is available at the time you want to take your refresher. Try to find something that stimulates you; you may feel that a course in neonatal intensive care, for example, will not be of great benefit to you as an independent practitioner, but it may be something that personally interests you. On the other hand, if this is the only course available, and it doesn't interest you, you may wish you'd booked earlier!

Insurance

Insurance is not just a matter of public liability and personal indemnity. You need to cover a lot of other things once you're in business for yourself.

Car

Car insurance is an important issue. Without your car you're stranded, so third party fire and theft probably isn't enough. Phone round, and get the cheapest fully comprehensive quote you can find, which includes business insurance. It won't cost you any extra.

Equipment

You also need to cover your equipment, both on the road and in the home. At home, the equipment is probably covered under the contents policy, but do make sure of this. If it isn't, insure it separately, or change your insurance policy. Insuring equipment on the road is slightly more difficult. The usual amount under your car insurance for property lost, stolen or destroyed in accident or fire is about £250. This will not go far. The Royal College of Midwives has details of companies who will insure equipment, but you can also try the big insurance brokers for comparison of price and facilities offered.

Professional insurance

As an individual, the midwife has three different levels of responsibility and, therefore, liability at law. The first area of responsibility which you have is purely as an individual. You have a personal duty of care to everybody. If you cause bodily injury, or physical damage, to the property of another by your negligence, or negligent behaviour, you have committed a 'tort'. As a 'tortfeasor' you may well be held liable for damages.

Third party liability

This liability can arise out of ownership of premises, for example, loose slates on a roof, or rickety stairs which can cause accidents to others; it can arise out of occupation of premises which you rent – carelessly discarded banana skins have made many lawyers rich. You can be negligent in the operation of a car when driving. This is why the Road Traffic Acts insist on motor insurance. Moreover, you could be responsible for the actions of your child, or dog, to say nothing about poking someone in the eye with an umbrella whilst walking down the street.

Obviously, the easiest way to avoid liability is never to put yourself at risk by being, at any time, negligent.

The insurance industry addresses the question of personal liability by providing cover, either alongside buildings insurance where you are the owner of property, or as part of the family of the owner of the building. If you rent accommodation, personal liability insurance is usually available when you arrange your contents insurance. Obviously, your car is insured; however, do take care that, when you drive someone else's car, it is insured for you to drive, and if you are going to use a boat, perhaps whilst on holiday, that proper insurance is in force before you do so. Cars and boats are normally excluded under a personal liability insurance, so you must always make sure of appropriate insurance for these activities.

Legal expenses

It is also worthy of note that many households buildings/contents insurance schemes now give the opportunity to purchase an extension for legal expenses. Most people with a job nowadays will find it very difficult to obtain significant legal aid for any action which they may wish to bring, against anyone else, for negligence. Legal expenses cover can give you a tool to exercise your rights, if you, yourself, feel that you need to pursue a claim against a third party.

Actions for damages

The next layer of liability arises from the actual practice of midwifery by a midwife. Obviously, you owe a duty of care to your client. Your client is entitled to rely on your professional ability. Perhaps the most important thing to remember is that an action for damages can be brought against you for up to 18 years after the birth. Some midwives believe their clients would never sue them because of the close relationship they have had with their client. This may be so in the short term. However, this memory may wear off and, confronted with the stark reality of injury to the mother and/or the child, compensation is not thought to be lightly dismissed.

The first line of defence is good practice. For a claim to succeed against you, it must be established that there was, in fact, negligence. Therefore, ensure that you adhere at all times to the Rules and Code of Practice, and, almost above all else, make sure that your paperwork is above reproach.

Until you become an independent practitioner and as long as you practice within the NHS on a contract, you have the benefit of vicarious liability. Whilst working under the NHS contract, the Regional Health Authority, in a master/servant relationship, assumed the liability for your acts. As an independent, you are in the front line. You must always remember that not only may you need a defence against a negligent act, error or omission, where such a thing has occurred, but it is possible to incur very high legal bills indeed, in defending an action against you, where you may be totally innocent of any alleged negligence.

Malpractice cover

One very important benefit which you receive as a member of the RCM is the malpractice liability cover which the College buys on behalf of its members. This indemnity used to be available to all midwives who are full members of the College, but is now only open to those who practice in an employed capacity, in either the NHS or the private sector. This effectively means that only those midwives who have no need of indemnity insurance have access to it, and that the only professional body catering solely for midwives chooses not to include those who may actually wish to make use of such cover!

Independents, who receive no reduction in their RCM subscriptions, have to make alternative arrangements if they wish to have malpractice cover. Whilst it is not a statutory requirement for midwives to carry such insurance, many midwives feel that, until there is a 'no-fault' compensation system, they have a moral duty to be insured. Others have made arrangements to put their house in the name of their partner or children and make sure that their clients know that they do not carry malpractice insurance. The reason for this is that, at the time of writing, the only insurance cover available to midwives practising independently is from the Medical Defence Union and, in 1997, costs £10,800 – as much as it costs to insure a consultant obstetrician.

The cost of insurance at the Royal College of Midwives is borne within the annual subscription, and the amount is currently set at £3 million for any one claim. The level of RCM cover is reviewed every year to keep pace with level of awards made by the courts and there is no limit on the MDU cover. It should be noted, however, that the MDU plans are for individual midwives and whilst a personal loan is available at a low rate of interest, this means that £1080 of your income per month will go on insurance costs so you need to cost this into your fees. Each midwife in the practice will need to be individually covered in her own right, so include all these fees if you are putting a business plan together.

You may be thinking of establishing a midwifery practice with another midwife, or opening midwifery clinics, or taking on a secretary. In this event, it could well be considered that the contract between the midwife and her client is not a personal one, but a contract between the practice and the client.

Joint practice cover

The practice in this case has no insurance cover, and it is a matter of great importance that this cover be obtained. Where there are employees, the midwifery practice itself becomes part of the master/servant relationship in the same way as the Health Authority protects its own employees. As an illustration, suppose your friend, working purely on a part-time basis, fails to pass on a crucial message about a woman in labour. If something dreadful happens, are you liable? Are you protected by your professional organization's cover?

It is possible that the woman's solicitors would advise her not to sue only you, but also the practice. You were not at fault. You had no means of knowing that the woman was about to go into labour; you may well have left detailed instructions regarding messages and phone calls, but, at the end of the day, you were unable to fulfil your contract. The negligent party was your employee who would be considered part of the practice.

Another scenario may run as follows: you are working on your own, but have naturally made arrangements for someone else to give emergency cover to your clients. In the event of your locum giving rise to a claim, it is perfectly possible that you yourself may be sued, as the contract was between you and the client. Your locum may benefit from college or union cover, but you will not, as the cover is for your acts as an individual. At the very least, you could be facing considerable legal bills before the 'deep pocket' is identified.

There are schemes which will cover independent midwives for practice insurance. Contact your insurance broker, or find a broker who specializes in this area. The MDU may be able to help or advise you.

Liability for employees

If you become an employer, you have a statutory duty to provide a safe working environment for your employees. You are also required to purchase employers liability insurance. If you decide to set up your practice from home, you must ensure that your premises are considered satisfactory from a safety point of view. You should also advise your home insurers that you are using your premises for professional purposes. In addition, it is possible (but not definite) that you may require planning permission. Your local council planning department will be able to advise you on this.

From all this, you will understand that your practice exposes you to risks. The first line of defence is careful practice, the back-up, plenty of insurance. This is a cost which should be incorporated in the fees which you charge. Do not forget to add the cost of protecting yourself, and your practice, into your business plan.

Summary

- Obtain copies of all UKCC documents, particularly the Rules and Code of Practice.
- Develop an extensive knowledge of the Rules and Code of Practice.
- Know your rights and responsibilities for continuing your professional education.
- Assess your needs for all types of insurance, and make sure you get a good deal.

CHAPTER THREE

Professional Issues

Drugs – supply, possession, administration and destruction

Do be sure to read the Rules and Code of Practice on this subject. More midwives have fallen over this hurdle than any other, so also refer to the UKCC's document on 'Standards for the Administration of Drugs' (1992).

CDAs

Many independent midwives do not carry pethidine for a variety of reasons. Some of these reasons are personal (for example, they may not wish to have Controlled Drugs of Addiction [CDAs] in their homes) and some professional (they are not convinced that the disadvantages of giving pethidine outweigh the advantages). If you decide to carry CDAs, the Code of Practice says you should seek advice from your Supervisor of Midwives 'regarding any matters related to the supply, administration, storage, surrender and destruction of CDAs and other medicines'. However, you should be prepared to keep your drugs in a separate, locked cupboard, and CDAs in a locked section inside that.

Pethidine can be obtained by asking for a supply order from your Supervisor. Alternatively, the woman can obtain her own supply from her GP. After she has delivered, any remaining pethidine should be destroyed, by her or her partner, as it is her property, while you watch. *You must record all transactions involving controlled drugs* – not least because your Supervisor has a right to audit those records.

Other medications

As a midwife, you also have the right to carry certain other medications: antiseptics, sedatives, analgesics, local anaesthetics, oxytocic preparations and 'approved agents for neonatal and maternal resuscitation'. This is powerful stuff, and you need to think carefully about what you need, and where and how you will store it all. The local Supervisor will advise you, and you can find out about these individual drugs from a pharmacist. The drugs themselves are listed in Schedule 3, parts 1 and 2 of the Medicines (products other than veterinary drugs) (prescription only) Order 1983 SI no. 1212, and any subsequent Orders. Within the framework of the Code of Practice, it is really up to you what drugs you would like to carry for your practice, but there are some which are more useful than others. You will also be expected to know the side effects and any contra-indications of those drugs. Vitamin K is a particular example; many parents will ask you for your advice, and you must be up to date on any and all advice that you give. Most independent midwives do not carry Vitamin K. There are two major reasons for this. The first is that it is not on the list of drugs that a midwife may carry – it must be prescribed, for that baby, by a doctor. The second is that, at the moment, there are no licensed oral preparations on the market. Consult your Supervisor on this matter.

Do remember that you must not use any medication, or any method of pain relief, until you have been trained in its use, and it has been approved by the Council for that use by midwives. TENS has now been approved by the UKCC, and some midwives like to carry their own. You could also rent out your TENS equipment if you're not likely to be using it for a while.

Premises or your home is not necessarily your castle

Right of inspection

Under certain circumstances, you may find that your privacy is not as inviolable as it was before you became an independent midwife. If you decide to use part, or all, of your home for professional purposes, you must be prepared for visitations. This means that you may decide to have clients visit your home, and use the spare bedroom as a consulting room. If you do, then the Supervisor, the relevant National Board and the Local Supervising Authority all have the right to inspect that part of your premises. It doesn't mean they have the right to look under your bed (unless you've been delivering clients in it), but they do have the right to go over your spare room with the aim of assessing its suitability for the purposes you propose.

If you have separate consulting rooms, or you have established a maternity home, then they have the right to inspect those premises in their entirety, and you will use your 'best endeavours to permit such an inspection to take place'. This means that even if you are not the manager of the home, you still have a responsibility to try to facilitate inspections by your Supervisor.

Places of antenatal visits

Where to do antenatal visits is a matter for each individual midwife to decide. You may prefer to visit the client's own home, or you may, perhaps because you have your own young children, suggest that clients visit you. It is worth planning do at least one visit to the client's home before she goes into labour. This is not a statutory requirement; it just means that, if she lives somewhere obscure, you have at least set eyes on the place before that 3 o'clock in the morning phone call.

Consulting rooms

If you decide to set up your own, separate consulting rooms, think about the following points.

1. Can you afford the initial outlay? If not, and you apply for a loan to cover the lease/rent, will you be able to repay it on the terms arranged? Will you have enough clients to bring in the income you will need? Are there any extras, such as business rates, ground rent, insurance, caretaking, heating, cleaning and so on?

2. Can you find someone to share the expense with you? Another independent midwife perhaps, or an alternative practitioner, such as a homeopath, for example?

3. You will need to charge extra to cover your overheads. Will the local market stand it? Will other independents in your area be charging less than you because they don't have your expenses?

4. You need to make sure that your consulting rooms are in an area which is easily accessible to your clients. Think about bus stops, car parking, stations. Pregnant women may not want to have to walk miles – is the street well lit, are the pavements adequate?

5. It is not a good idea to have your consulting rooms on the fourth floor of a building with no lift. This can play havoc with accurate recording of your clients' blood pressure.

6. You need to have more than just a room. You will need a lavatory for clients (and you) to use, and somewhere to wash your hands. You may also want somewhere to make tea or coffee, and perhaps a small fridge. All these need to be kept scrupulously clean – who will do the domestic tasks?

7. If you intend that an office will form part of your consulting rooms, how secure will it be? You will be keeping confidential information there, and possibly expensive equipment. The equipment can be

insured, but the information will be irreplaceable. Losing information can lose you your reputation.

8.   Is any furniture supplied, or will you have to buy it in? It's all very well thinking about an examination couch, a desk, or a computer, but what about tissues, loo rolls, and gel for the fetal stethoscope? How will you make the place look pretty and welcoming all the time? Who will buy the plants or flowers? Is there a phone? Who will act as receptionist, and answer the phone if you have to leave suddenly to go to a birth?

9.   Do not pay out any money until you have discussed the potential consulting rooms with a Supervisor.

Consulting rooms need a lot of thought.

Gathering the right tools for the job

Your equipment represents a major capital investment. Don't rush out and buy the first pair of Kochers forceps that you see. There may well be cheaper ones elsewhere, and, anyway, Kochers may not do the job as well as Spencer-Wells.

Make a list of what you need *just to start*. It will probably include all your antenatal bits and pieces, and should contain at least the following articles.

Antenatal equipment
- Portable doppler fetal heart detector.
- Pinard stethoscope (for when the above's battery runs out).
- Sphygmomanometer – the small digital ones work well antenatally, but are not so reliable in labour. Moving targets give a false reading.
- Stethoscope – a cheap one is just as good as the more expensive ones.
- Urine testing sticks – antenatally, you really only need to test for protein and glucose, but you may like to choose more extensive ones for use in labour.
- Tape measure, if you are accustomed to using one.
- Venepuncture equipment:
    – tourniquet
    – syringes and needles, or vacutainers
    – blood bottles
    – test request cards
    – container to keep it all in.
- Plastic folders for notes.
- Bag to carry all this.

The labour and postnatal list is longer. Buy what you feel to be the essentials first. In addition to the above, you will need:

Birthing equipment
- Sterile gloves.
- Thermometer.
- Inco pads.
- Entonox/oxygen and cylinder heads.
- Instruments, which should include:
  - Spencer Wells or Kochers forceps x 2
  - pair of large, sharp scissors
  - pair of suture scissors
  - stitch holder
  - dissecting forceps
  - speculum for high vaginal swabs (you can get disposable ones).

Sterilization
Some sort of sterilizeable container with a well fitting lid; heavy duty plastic is as good as stainless steel. Keep the sterilized instruments in this. You can boil your instruments for twenty minutes, then using sterile tongs, put them in the sterilized container. If your tongs and container are plastic, you can sterilize them in solution while the instruments are boiling. Alternatively, you can autoclave your instruments at the local health centre or hospital, if you ask nicely. You may have to pay a small fee. Keep them double wrapped in a sterile cloth (tea towels or muslin nappies are ideal), and paper until you need them.

Disposables
- Syringes and needles.
- Sharps disposal container.
- Sterile mucous extractors – double chamber.
- Cotton wool packs, sterile and ordinary.
- Sterile gauze swabs.
- Urinary catheters (non-retaining).
- Sanitary towels.
- Suture material.
- Sterile cord clamps.
- Amnihook.
- Inco pads.

Drugs

- Pethidine.
- Syntometrine.
- Ergometrine.
- Local anaesthetic.
- Local treatment for haemorrhoids.
- Glycerine suppositories.
- Disinfectant hand cleanser – don't forget, you will have to pay for all these.

Lotion

- Transducer gel.
- Some sort of lubricant (be aware that many women are sensitive to obstetric cream).
- Lotions, for vulval swabbing etc. (you may like to try the natural based lotions, such as Calendula tincture for antisepsis, and arnica or hammamelis for relief of perineal symptoms).

Postnatal equipment

- Baby scales (anglers spring balances are easy to carry, pretty accurate and cheap).
- Umbilical cord tape.
- Lancets for Guthrie tests etc.
- Cards for Guthrie Tests, serum bilirubin.
- Capillary tubes for serum bilirubin.
- A good camera.
- A heavy duty, bright torch.

Emergency equipment

For emergencies, you'll need the following:

- Oxygen, maternal and neonatal.
- Laryngoscope, with infant blade.
- Laerdal bag and mask.
- Airways – adult and neonatal.
- IV catheter and giving set, with some sticky plaster.
- IV fluid (1 litre Hartmann's solution, followed by 0.5 litre gelufusin is the recommended emergency regime for a haemorrhage. It is vitally important that you are taught to insert an IV catheter. Putting up an IV while veins are still patent can save your client's life).

Containers

You may like to keep the maternal and baby emergency equipment in two separate boxes. Plastic tool boxes with compartments inside do a perfect job. This will give you space to include items such as emergency blood bottles, syringes and needles and sterile gloves. You can use double-sided sticky patches to hold everything in place and stop it rolling about. Do remember that because you use these things (hopefully) very rarely, if at all, you will need to check them at regular intervals to make sure they're not out of date.

Bags

The bags you buy to carry all your equipment need to be light, but strong and made of some wipe-clean material. Have as many pockets and sections as you are likely to need, as you will have papers to carry in addition to the rest the kit. Shoulder straps are a boon. Nobody has yet found a convenient way of carrying two entonox cylinders, so you should realize that you are unlikely to be able to carry all your gear into the house in one trip, unless you have help.

Expensive extras

When you do have some spare money, you may like to think about a few extras, for example:

- Your own TENS equipment.
- Your own portable birth pool.
- Your own suction equipment.

Purchasing equipment

As for stockists, be wary. Many of the equipment suppliers are very expensive, and you can easily find that some suppliers are cheaper than others. Ask other independents what they carry; you could also ask them (cautiously) if they're thinking of retiring – if they are, you could offer to buy the equipment. This doesn't happen often. The Secretary of the IMA may know of any independents who are giving up, so ask her before you spend any money. If you have a contact at your local hospital, ask them if they have any spare/old (but functioning) equipment they would be willing to let you buy. You can also buy your stocks of disposables from the local hospital. Their prices will be very competitive, and they tend not to run out of stock just when you want some cotton wool balls.

Some companies, particularly those selling oxygen and entonox equipment, may have reconditioned offers, often for a fraction of the new price. Do phone around before you decide. Always ask for a professional discount, even from the local pharmacist; you may not get one, but it's worth asking.

Alternative remedies

There may also be special things that you want to use, such as homeopathic remedies or aromatherapy oils. Do make sure that you have received adequate training in their use, or you could find yourself in trouble.

Lastly, remember that you will have to cart this lot about. Lightweight bags and plastic containers will ease your load considerably, and so will only taking with you what is necessary for that birth!

Phones and pagers

You will also need a form of communication which enables you to leave home for periods longer than five minutes. A pager, or, if you're rich, a mobile phone will serve the purpose. If you don't have a pager of some sort, you can bet that someone will need to contact you desperately just when you've nipped up the road for a paper. There are numerous schemes for different sorts of pagers and phones. You can buy, rent or lease. You can have varying amounts of coverage in terms of area. You can have tone or message pagers. Decide what is likely to be most useful and phone every company in the book. You could also ask other independents which they use, and why. Most independents use a message pager rather than a tone one, as this tells them immediately who is trying to contact them, and whether it's urgent or not. A few have mobile phones. It is likely that as the price of operating these comes down, they will become increasingly popular.

Answerphones

An answerphone is another vital piece of equipment. Without it, you have no idea who has tried to ring you, and failed, or how many clients you have lost because they weren't able to talk to you. Most telecommunications companies sell answerphones, or you can rent one for a reasonable price from British Telecom. It is worth investing in a Mercury line for your long distance calls – this will help to reduce your phone bill, as will only making long distance calls after 6pm wherever possible. If you are in an area where cable companies are putting in phone lines, then investigate this. Local calls are often free at certain times and this will save a great deal of money.

Office equipment

You should have a typewriter or a word processor. Often there are bargains to be found in used computer shops, or the small ads column of the local paper. Handwritten letters are fine for your family (and probably mandatory for any Great Aunts), but they won't do in the business world. Typing is a skill which improves with repetition, even if you only ever use the two fingered method. If you have a word processor, or a personal computer, get the best printer you can afford. This may be second hand, or reconditioned. You can set up your word processor to print your letter heads, which will save you money on your stationery, and you can keep copies of all your documents on disc which will save considerable space.

Transport

You need reliable transport. If you are only intending to cover a small local area, a bike might do – with a large carrier for the equipment – but most independents need a motorized form of transport. Do have your car regularly serviced; this usually means you don't get nasty surprises in the small hours of the morning when it won't start. It also makes it cheaper to run. Find a garage who knows how important your car is to you, and who will arrange a loan car for you when yours is in dock. Lastly, make sure you always have enough petrol in the car to go to the next birth. This may sound self evident, but you may be called to see her as an emergency, rather than when she is in labour, so never let the fuel go over the red line. All night garages can be few and far between when you really need one.

To sum up, whether you are buying a thermometer or a car, don't buy the first one you see; use the phone to check prices, it saves a lot of travelling; don't think institutional, think, 'Do I really need it, and, if I do, will plastic do the job as well?'. In short – making business decisions starts here.

Honorary contracts – searching for the Grail

As a rule, most independent midwives support homebirths as the prime option for healthy women having a normal pregnancy. Having said that, however, women have been brainwashed for the last forty years into believing that the safest place for them to have babies is a hospital. It sometimes amazes me that so many women are able to fight this conditioning and insist on homebirths. We are slowly but surely seeing the incidence of homebirths increase, but until it is viewed as a normal option by the majority of women, we are going to need a facility which enables clients to deliver in hospital with an independent as their choice of midwife. Domino deliveries are an exciting alternative for many women.

Continuity of carer is often more important to women than place of birth, and many independents see this continuity as an opportunity to encourage women to make informed choices about their place of birth. It can be difficult to talk in any depth to people you have never seen before, and may never see again. This is part of the difficulty facing many women in the hospital system, who would like to discuss their wishes, have their fears reassured and their hopes supported. The GPs, who are often the point of most continuity for women, are almost universally opposed to homebirth, so the safety and reality of choice is never stated.

Given the factors militating against homebirth, we cannot expect to change attitudes overnight. It will take some time. Therefore, for the time being, there are going to be women who want your service, but who are not ready yet to contemplate having their baby at home. So, you need an honorary contract. These can take many diverse forms (sometimes, literally). You may get a contract which permits you to have access to labour ward in order to deliver your client. It may say that in case of an abnormality developing, you will contact the medical staff on call. This is probably the best sort of contract to have. It has the virtue of brevity, and doesn't say anything about following hospital policies. If, in order to get a contract, you have to sign one which says you will follow hospital policy, it is a good thing to remember that you cannot do anything to which your client doesn't consent. If she doesn't want you to rupture her membranes, well, what can you do? If she isn't following the labour ward protocols on progress in labour, unless it constitutes an abnormality, you and she must decide what is the best course to follow – nobody else. There are usually ways round these restrictive covenants.

Who to ask

Your Supervisor is the person who probably organizes these contracts for you, although sometimes, particularly in Trust hospitals, she may feel the need to contact the management committee. It should be stressed by her that you are providing women with a valid choice, and if for no other reason, you should receive a contract on that basis. Life is not always fair though, and you may be refused. If possible, get the reasons for your refusal in writing, then you can try to appeal against it. Write to the executive committee, and ask them why they won't give you a contract when GPs, consultants and dentists get them. Refer them to the NHS Management Executive document on private practice in NHS hospitals for confirmation. Talk to the Supervisor, and ask her what she thinks is the problem. She may be able to help you formulate a response which may win the day. Contact the Community Health Council and explain the problem; talk to local consumer groups and see if you can enlist their support.

If none of this works, then turn your attention to another hospital. There are usually alternatives, unless you work in a very rural area. You could, if this is indeed your situation, try to negotiate a deal which says that, in an emergency, you could accompany your clients into hospital and provide their care. This may serve as the thin end of the wedge for you. If everything fails, then wait six months and try again.

Summary

- Open discussions with local Supervisors.
- Be aware of all regulations and information concerning the drugs you use.
- Choose which drugs and medications you intend to use.
- Draft an equipment list, and phone around for the best deal.
- Decide whether you are intending to have consulting rooms.
- Commence negotiations for honorary contracts.

CHAPTER FOUR

Money Matters

Banking and accounting
Starting a small business

You are now considering starting a small business. You may have thought that you were just 'going independent', but it ain't that simple. You now have to view yourself as a businesswoman – at least, you do if you want to eat. Even if you have a rich partner, you will, presumably, still want to earn some money from your practice. You have to be business minded about your financial affairs. After all, you still have to pay tax and National Insurance, so it makes sense to claim every last penny to which you are entitled.

Visit any High Street bank and get a copy of their small business pack. The packs go on and on about writing a business plan, how to project cash flow, and calculating profit and loss accounts. This may, naturally, be supremely interesting to you, but will it be useful? The most useful aspect of the small business packs are the advice they give to people starting up in business for themselves for the first time. If you are intending to ask the bank for a loan (see below), they may ask you for a business plan, but otherwise you can take a great deal of time and trouble writing something which is of no use whatsoever.

You need a separate business account. Open this account as soon as you make the decision to start independent practice. Think carefully about where you want this account to be. Do you want it at your existing bank, or can you get a better deal elsewhere? Most banks will give you a first year free from bank charges, but will there be interest payable when you are in credit? How much will that interest be? What about the Post Office, or a building society – how do they compare? When you have set up your business account, pay all your fees and payments into it, and pay yourself a salary, into your personal account, from it.

Finding funding

The initial costs of setting up in practice can be difficult to meet. This can be arranged with your bank, either as an overdraft, or as a personal loan if you don't have that sort of cash in your account. Do not rely on getting the overdraft, *or* the loan until you have it in writing.

There is also the Prince's Youth Business Trust, but only if you are under 30. Unless you have St Jude for a bank manager, or you already have security, such as unmortgaged property, don't even bother to ask for a small business loan. An overdraft facility can be a possibility, though, for buying equipment, and so on.

Book keeping and accounting

You need to have at least a book keeper, if not an accountant, unless this is a skill you already possess. Keep all your receipts, for everything, and write down every payment you receive. You will be amazed at how much is tax deductible.

If you don't keep receipts, you stand to lose money that you might have been able to claim back from the tax man. Then give the whole lot, at regular intervals, to your book keeper. This service will cost you from about £6 an hour. It's worth it.

Your book keeper will organize your tax affairs for you, and prepare your books to be approved by an accountant. As a self employed person, you can claim for all sorts of things. The tax office will not do this for you, so you need someone who can. Personally, I feel the hassle of sorting out the Inland Revenue is a specialist job for which I am more than happy to pay. You may enjoy the challenge.

Getting used to charging

One of the most difficult issues to deal with in independent practice is that of asking for money for your services. It takes a lot of practice before you become comfortable with this idea. The idea of charging a small amount which every woman can reasonably afford seems fine when you have a salary each month. Out in the less sheltered world of self-employment, it soon becomes obvious that you have to charge a reasonable amount just to be able to pay your bills. However, you don't just want to pay the bills. You want to go on holiday, buy extravagant underwear, take a friend to lunch – life isn't only about the necessities. It also seems reasonable to assume that you have a marketable commodity. You've trained and worked for years to get to this point. Why undervalue yourself, and, incidentally, every other independent midwife, by charging an inadequate amount?

As midwives, and as women, we seem to be rather bad at setting a monetary value on what we do. We may see ourselves as asking for money for what is popularly perceived as a free service. People tend to forget that they are already paying for the NHS through National Insurance. If doctors, dentists, physiotherapists and a multitude of others can offer their services outside the NHS, so can we! In order to overcome this diffidence, be confident that you are offering something very special. You are giving a personal service, individually tailored for each client. Be proud of what you do, and it won't seem so bad when you say the amount you charge out loud (see the section in Chapter 5 'Changing your self image').

Extra contractual referrals (ECRs)

There have been instances when a woman has been unable to obtain appropriate care from her local NHS. This tends to happen when a woman wants a mode of care which is out of the mainstream, for example, a birth at home. Although authorities have a clear obligation under the NHS Act to provide this service, some have refused to do so 'except in an emergency'. Under these special circumstances, the woman has contacted local independents who have undertaken her care. The woman has then billed the district health authority to cover the independents' invoice. On those occasions when the bill has been met, this has been on the grounds that the DHA has an obligation to provide care, and they have failed to do so (see also the section 'Tendering to Health Authorities').

Pricing it right

Payment schedules

Don't expect to receive your fees in a lump sum. This is difficult for most people, and in any case, it helps your cashflow to have your payments in regular instalments. Document the arrangement for paying (in the notes, if you like) and you and your client should both sign it to say that these arrangements are satisfactory to you both. Most independents like to have all the money paid before the due date, but occasionally you may have a client who needs a longer time to pay.

You need to decide what you are going to charge. *Do* be realistic. You can't live on £6 an hour, even if book keepers do. They have more clients per day. At the moment, the sensible rate seems to be £30–50 an hour, which means a total fee, per client, of between £1200 and £2500. Be aware that most independents are prepared to negotiate fees. It may make you feel very uncomfortable to turn a client away because she can't afford your services; some women may need longer to pay, or perhaps you may be prepared to offer a discount. In some cases, you may like to discuss a bartering system – one midwife had her kitchen fitted in lieu of payment! Once you have accepted the principle that your time and skills have a value, think about other aspects of what you do. Consultations are an example, when people want to talk to you before they make a decision. This can take quite a lot of time, often in the evenings when you can meet the woman and her partner together. If you charge £30 as your consultation fee, you can then explain to the woman that this will be deducted from the full amount if she decides to book you. Otherwise you could find yourself seriously out of pocket, when you take your time and travelling expenses into account. You may also be asked to do lectures and talks to student midwives, refresher courses and so on. Charge appropriately for your time – your hourly rate will be quite acceptable. If you are asked for interviews, or to write articles, again always ask about a fee. If there is no fee payable, the publicity may be worth going without a fee – but then again it may not! Use your judgement.

Budgeting

You need to assess how much money you are going to pay yourself, and how much you need for business expenses. The latter is tax deductible, the former is not. Legitimate business expenses include such things as disposable items, other professional fees (for example, for cover from a midwife, or for your book keeper), advertising, and so on. Allow a budget wherever possible, especially with regard to advertising, and if you're not getting a response to a particular form, then stop doing it. Nothing wastes money faster than ineffective advertising. Do consult with your financial adviser especially over tax matters.

Safety in (birth) numbers

Client planning

You need to decide what is the optimum number of clients you can manage on a monthly basis. Most independents practising singlehanded feel that two deliveries in a four week period is about right. The last thing you need when you are happily rubbing a clients back, safe in the knowledge that she is eight centimetres dilated and everything is going well, is a call on your pager to say that you are needed urgently by another client. So, space your clients well, and in all cases do make sure that they know what to do in case you are, by some unhappy stroke of fate, with another client or have fallen under a bus. It is important to let clients know that even if they have booked your services, they are still entitled to all the usual NHS care, and can still have access to NHS midwives and care if you are, for whatever reason, unavailable.

If you are setting up a partnership, or a group practice then the figures can be slightly different. You can still book two each in a four week period, but you will probably be safe to add another one to that. This means that for two partners you can take five clients, for three partners seven etc.

If you take two clients a month, on full fees, this will net you roughly £2500 a month. It sounds a lot when taken in the abstract, but remember that if there are two or three of you in the practice, then £2500 doesn't go that far. Also, some months you may not have any bookings at all, so the money you earned in previous months will have to last you.

Writing a business plan

If you are applying for a loan, or trying to get financial support for a pet scheme, then you will certainly be asked to write a business plan. These are roughly divided into two sections – the words and the numbers. The words should incorporate the background for your idea, why it is a good idea, the germ of the idea itself, and how you see it progressing in the future. The numbers will include estimated profit and loss, projected cash flow, costs of absolutely everything you are likely to need, and should indicate clearly the amount you need to start up the scheme, and how/when it will be repaid.

You can get pre-prepared business plans in the small business packs available from any high street bank, but these tend to talk about sales and stock, which is not applicable to the type of business that you are likely to be contemplating. It's actually better to write your own, because then you can adapt the plan to your specific needs. There is an example of a business plan in Appendix 5 but you'll have to put in your own figures. You can make the business plan as long as you like, but remember that financial people are likely to read the figures first, and, only if they find those interesting, will they turn to the text. Take advice from people experienced in the field – business managers usually have a good idea of what's effective, and what will be perceived as waffle. Make it as professional as you can; have it printed nicely (ask a friend with a laser printer) and bound at a printshop. Take several copies – people don't always send them back – and be prepared to kiss a lot of toads before you meet the handsome prince.

Summary

- Open a business account.
- Plan your client numbers.
- Practise discussing the fee you will charge.
- Assess the need for a business plan.
- Consider tendering to local GPs, hospitals etc.

CHAPTER FIVE

Marketing Yourself

Getting into the traffic

When you first set up your own business, one of the most common problems is that you begin to feel rather isolated. Making the effort to 'get into the traffic' is another way of saying that staying at home on your own will not gain you any business, any contacts, any new information, any lucky breaks; you have to be visible, be out 'there' to make things happen. This is advocated by all of the business gurus and it makes a lot of sense. Successful people aren't found holed away in their studies, not returning phone calls and keeping the mileage down on their cars. They are out at every opportunity. They are visible to those people who may wish to use their services, in other words, they are on the market and the consumer can see that.

Obviously, there is more to being 'in the traffic' than just out of the house. In order to create and take advantage of new opportunities to learn, to win new clients, to obtain help and advice from those who have something valuable to offer, you have to be in the right places.

Being in the right place

With a target client base of women wanting midwifery services, it is easy to see that you need to be around women, particularly those who are more likely to be pregnant or to be close to someone who is having a baby. You are part of a local community that offers facilities and services to women – find out what they are and become part of that activity. Sources of information for these group activities include schools, church/community centres, medical practices, local newspapers and notice boards, libraries and shopping centres.

It should not be forgotten that there will also be a large group of men who should also be targeted – those who want only the best for their partners and new babies and could be convinced to invest in an independent midwife. These will be men that are unlikely to be found in a pool hall but may well be part of other types of group activity; perhaps sports centres, cricket clubs or professional associations. They may be located at work so find out about public notice boards in company buildings or ask someone you know who works in one to put the notice up for you.

Be creative in your attempts to get into the traffic. The more people you mix with, the more chance you will have of meeting those who will want to make the choice to use your services or those who will pass that information on to others who may be interested. Be lateral in your thinking; maternity groups are not the only place you will find your leads.

Keep a diary

Keep records of places you go, groups you meet, people you get to know by name, opportunities you may spot that you can follow up later, contacts you make who might be useful, sources of information or help that were especially good – all of this information will help you to get ahead. You will do a lot of 'leg work' to begin with, so record everything so that the lessons you learn early on will not be wasted later.

Networking

You may wish to share this information with other midwives; of course, this will encourage them to share their experiences with you, so it is valuable exchange. This is what is known as networking, a relatively new name for a process that has been happening in all walks of life for centuries! What might be newer to you is the idea that networking will actually be a source of business ideas and contacts for you, so think of it as a valuable part of your working life. You may wish to do this more formally in writing, through a newsletter for example, especially if you find this easier to organize and you have the facilities to produce it. You do not have to restrict it to other midwives; indeed, you may find it broadens your horizons and adds new dimensions to what you can achieve if you include in your informal or formal network people who run other kinds of small business or consultancies.

Current trends

Whether or not you become involved in any PR activities for midwives (see later section), it is important to keep up with what is happening in the world of clients, so read women's magazines (they will get some of their information and form opinions based on these), read local newspapers for information about local events and issues that will matter to the clients, watch local news programmes on television especially any programmes related to birth, listen to radio programmes such as Radio 4's Women's Hour – all of these sources will keep you up to date with what is important to other women. Your opinion is your own, but at least be informed on the issues your target clients will be involved with, as this will help you to understand them better and know where to find them and how to reach them. Large agencies call this market research and spend hundreds of thousands of pounds keeping in touch with what people want and think and feel and do, so that they can target them for them for sales campaigns.

Changing your self image

As a midwife, you offer a high level of professional care to women in various stages of childbirth. As a business person, you are selling your services to consumers. The transition from carer to salesperson is psychologically a difficult one to achieve. Once you can really see yourself as a business, with a product/service to sell, profits to make and bills to pay, you will be a long way further down the road to success, on your terms. Once you have defined your goals in terms of what you want to achieve in your business and set yourself an action plan to reach those targets, you will need to be able to change your self-image to accommodate your change in status.

One of the hardest aspects of working for yourself is being able to charge what seems like large amounts of money for what you do. Almost every consultant experiences this, but women find it particularly difficult to ask for money for their services, for lots of reasons. Whatever the reason, you need to find a way to be very comfortable with the concept that you are worth £XXX and not have trouble facing up to telling people that, looking them straight in the eye as you do it. Remember all the builders, lawyers, accountants, plumbers and electricians that have looked you in the eye and told their charges – steel yourself and do the same!

An image of quality

Whatever you charge, you are competing with what is perceived as a free service, so you will need to offer clients a service that is clearly of the highest quality and involves a great level of care and attention. These will be among the features of your service; they need to be presented to the client along with the benefits of these features (what this means to the consumer, specifically how she will benefit).

Your clients will have in their minds some ideas about how a quality service should be presented – these values may vary from your ideas considerably. My idea of a good dentist, for example, involves him not asking about my holiday when I have a mouth full of sharp metal implements. In fact, I don't need the chat at all, it does not relax me or make me more confident that he is not merely making valuable work for himself by drilling holes in my teeth. What I need is to have a detailed understanding of exactly what is happening and how quickly it will all be over! I also require him never to eat garlic; the smell makes me feel quite ill.

Whether or not it is reasonable for me to expect my dentist not to eat garlic, I make my buying decision partly on this criterion. Your potential clients will have their own ideas about how you should look, smell and sound and what you should wear, drive and so on. Some of these things will probably agree with; not turning up at someone's house or clinic in black rubber suits or dirty overalls, for example. Some things you will not be prepared to compromise for the sake of the business; I will not work for companies that I consider to be 'unethical' (my judgement). You may not be prepared to dress in any other way than in your favourite, comfy tracksuit. You and only you can decide on how far you will go to present a professional image, as perceived by the general public. Be aware that you cannot force people to accept you the way you are if you can't get past their front door because your appearance or manner is unacceptable to them

Defining the product

Decide on how you want to appear to your consumers; how your 'product' will be 'packaged'. Then outline just what the consumer will get for the money you will charge and how many benefits you can find in your service. Be clear about what 'extras' you can offer within your resources of time, money and availability. Do not make an offer that cannot be fulfilled.

This product information will form the basis of all your marketing efforts.

SWOT analysis

Although it sounds complicated, this is just an analysis of your Strengths, Weaknesses, Opportunities and Threats. To an interior design company, I once presented these as Walls, Cracks, Windows and Stones, which is a more visual way of understanding this element of your business. You may not be able to fill in much detail under these categories at first, but certainly you will know your strengths (anything from 'I'm a good listener' to 'I can get to the Isle of Skye at a moment's notice') and may be able to get someone to help you with your weaknesses ('I don't drive' or 'I am not available in the afternoons when the children are home'). Your opportunities list will grow with time and experience, as you 'get into traffic'. Your threats are those things which might take your business away or threaten the way you operate. People tend to see threats as competition but it may be other things entirely, such as being under-capitalized.

The point about a SWOT analysis is that it helps you to understand your business better, plug those weaknesses, make features out of the strengths, seek more opportunities and be aware of the threats. It will help you target your marketing efforts accordingly.

Planning for success

The key to successful marketing lies in excellent planning and a disciplined approach to stick to those plans. A marketing plan is, in any case, a requirement for a business plan, should you need to borrow money from the bank to fund the early days when you have no income, or to buy a more reliable car. Plans can always be amended or even abandoned for new plans, but there is a saying 'Fail to plan and you plan to fail' that makes a lot of sense.

Setting goals

In order to market yourself successfully, you will need to set some realistic goals about what targets your business should reach. Add into the equation the money and time you will be able to allocate to marketing and this will enable you to write an action plan that is attainable and productive. If you do not set goals, your efforts will be more random, and you are likely to waste more time and money; ultimately, this will prove frustrating.

Action planning

Marketing depends on a lot of effort and this takes time – your time. This is the time that you are not seeing clients, shopping, picking up the children, cooking or cleaning or any of those other things that you need to do. Sometimes it will be sitting down in the evening and going through papers or magazines, researching your market, sometimes it may mean daytime hours in a local college business centre, designing a leaflet on the desktop publishing system. This time needs to be planned, otherwise the marketing jobs will simply not get done.

When you have set your business goals, allocated some money for marketing and decided how you wish to spend it, your next step is to write an action plan, otherwise known as a list or, in time management programmes, a Critical Path Analysis. It comes to the same thing; breaking down each action, such as 'produce a leaflet', into smaller steps, in this case, 'write copy, design the layout, produce artwork, phone three printers for quotes, take it to the printer, collect leaflets'. Of course, your list might involve asking other people to do these things for you, so your action is to make sure they do it! Set yourself dates by which step has to be done and stick to these; your marketing will stay on course if you follow your plans.

Monitoring success

When you have placed your small ad/delivered your leaflets/put your poster on the clinic wall, you will start to get some response. Make sure you know where each enquiry has come from (word of mouth/contact at coffee morning/clinic poster etc.) and note it against your marketing plan, so that you know what works and what does not work. Clearly the things that do not work should be a lower priority for further work than those things that did make an impact.

You will need to be ruthless with yourself about following up every contact, however tenuous, and checking your leaflets have been received or posters have not been ripped down a day later. Noting your successes will also help to motivate you to carry on with the effort!

Stepping into your customer's shoes

Just as you have had to take an objective view of yourself and your services, so you need to be more analytical about your target client. In order to decide how to persuade her to buy your services, you need to put yourself in her shoes, try to think as she might think and project yourself into her life. Imagine that she has no idea that such a thing as an independent midwife even exits to start with. Focus on what she might want to know, what information (or misinformation) she may have already received about midwifery services available to her. What does she read or watch? What other services might she buy – an interior designer, a gardener? Where do her children go to school? Where does she shop?

By putting yourself into her shoes, you can begin to target your marketing more effectively, answering the questions she would ask, giving her reassurance on the things that may concern her, being seen in the places where she goes. Many small business people assume that their clients will be like-minded people; this is not always the case. She may have different values, she will certainly have different experiences; you will need to be open to these in your marketing.

Summary

You should now have:

- A changed outlook on yourself and your business opportunities.
- A clear idea of your image and qualities.
- An idea of how to market those.
- A plan and a budget to achieve this.
- A clearer view of your target clients and how to reach them within your resources.

Putting the word out

Communication

Being seen in the marketplace is all very well, but the way you choose to communicate makes all the difference to your success rate. Marketing is largely based on principles of effective communicating.

In order to help the consumer to choose your services, you need to convey all the relevant information as well as be persuasive that the features you describe will have benefits for the consumer. The KISS principle is a good rule of thumb – Keep It Simple, Stupid! In other words, be clear, be precise, keep it brief, don't clutter your space, and use design to make the information easy to take in. Remember to be very positive in your tone, too. A good way to judge the success of anything you write or design is to ask someone who knows little about your business to read it through and give you an honest opinion about it. Ask if it is clear, repetitive, dull, friendly, informative – and whether it would lead to a further enquiry being made.

Quality in production

Maintain a quality approach, it does make a difference. If you can't afford to have something printed on quality paper, promise yourself you will save up for it, find a cheaper deal with a printer and in the meantime photocopy your artwork, if you must. You will be creating an overall impression that will be associated with your service.

Marketing tools

Business cards

This is the minimum you require – you must have something to leave with people that enables them to contact you later. So if this is the only thing you do, make sure it is professionally produced, imaginative, larger than a 'normal' card, more than one colour – something that people will want to keep.

The norm is to have a flat card with your name, address and phone number but you can vary this for a little extra cost – for example, have a 'tent card', which is twice the size folded in half and stands up by someone's phone or on a desk or sideboard. It has more space for information, such as when you are available in the area, or your radio-pager number, if you have one. You can be more creative with a design that will create a good impression, such as one that shows you as being very caring or very professional.

Leaflets

These are also cheap to produce, usually A4 folded into three (gatefold) or in half. Be wary of the printer using very cheap, lightweight, white paper, as this will have a very disposable feel to the recipient – you want it to be kept. Ask to see paper samples and choose something not glossy, around 135-150 gsm (grams per square metre) in weight, in an ivory or natural white rather than bright white, or a pale colour if you like. Having photographs reproduced increases the cost quite significantly, but line drawings are treated more or less as text. Keep the drawings or graphics simple as well, so that they enhance the overall impression, rather than cluttering the space and detracting from the text.

The idea of having a leaflet is that it is very flexible, it gives lots of room to explain your features and benefits, plus you can use plenty of space to make the contact details very clear and bold. Leaflets can be left in public places for people to pick up (they do), or put through letterboxes, pinned to notice boards or handed to someone in person.

Posters

Posters really make an impact, if you can find sites to put them up. You can also be really imaginative in your design – try a local art college for students to design one for you, to a strict brief about information it must convey. The other advantage is that they are seen repeatedly by the public, who then know where to look when they have a need for you services, or they will pass the information on.

The printing of posters is usually better done by a screenprinter (see your local phone book) or if you are feeling creative, most colleges run evening classes in screenprinting! The same college might have students who could print them for you, for a low rate. The advantage of screenprinting is that you can print as few or as many as you need, unlike offset litho printing, which is a rapid machine process with larger cost-effective quantities.

Personal canvassing

By telephone or on foot, personal calls are expensive in terms of your time, so this is recommended only as a follow up to another type of campaign, such as leaflet distribution or a poster in a place with limited local viewers. This also requires a large dollop of self confidence; not for the faint hearted.

Creative promotions

Marketing can involve some wonderfully creative ideas. An event of some kind is often successful – an open evening, say, at which you can talk to a group about the opportunities available to them through your services, allay any fears and offer advice. You might promote this by taking round balloons with 'Birth Day' on them, perhaps, to pregnant women on a local GP's register.

Advertising and public relations (PR) are dealt with in a later section.

Agencies and alternatives

Advertising or marketing agencies may be available to you locally, but you are unlikely to be able to afford their services.

Printers often offer a design service, but this is usually very limited. If you can give them a good idea of what you want, they will not offer much in the way of creativity but will be able to follow clear instructions. Sometimes, they might employ the services of a graphic artist, in which case you are better off doing this directly.

Students at your local art college may be persuaded to do work for you for very low rates. Try contacting a Head of Department especially if they cover graphic design, rather than fine art.

Colleges also run short part-time courses or evening classes in some areas of design; this might be more cost-effective than hiring someone to do it for you, plus you have long term benefit of being able to design for more than one project.

Some colleges also have small business centres, which will have the computer design facilities that may be adequate for your needs. Remember that courses as well as your design/printing costs are tax deductable.

Summary

- You should now have enough information to try some of these ideas.
- Research contacts who might offer help.
- Find out about facilities near you.
- Decide what to include in your marketing plan and set yourself an action plan with deadlines.

Engaging media interest

Public relations

Public relations (PR) is, broadly speaking, the pursuit of public exposure through unpaid appearances or free reporting of your story, rather than paid for advertising space. It might include sending out press releases on a specific news story related to independent midwifery; appearing on a radio chat show as a guest speaker; an unpaid speech at a dinner or luncheon; handing out prizes at a local school function or writing letters to the editors of newspapers or magazines.

Free publicity

This is often regarded as 'free publicity', but in terms of your time, you will find it anything but 'free'. Often the exposure you can obtain is worth the effort; you can reach far more women in need of your services through a radio programme than you could afford with a mailshot. Some PR may only raise awareness at a very general level ('Oh, I never knew midwives could practise independently!') and not lead to any actual business in a directly quantifiable way. The rules of thumb are to be as involved in any PR opportunity as you can afford to be; group monitoring of these opportunities is usually far more successful than individual efforts and it is definitely who you know that counts!

If you do decide to run a PR campaign, remember it is personal contacts you need to develop and nurture, as well as writing good copy/press releases/stories, taking every photo opportunity (black and white print for newspapers, colour transparency for magazines) and religiously keeping press cuttings and relevant stories from other sources. When you do get your big chance to appear/speak/write, you need a barrage of facts, figures, real life examples and supporting information at your fingertips, so be prepared, keep your library up to date.

Handling the media

Not only will it be hard work to develop media contacts, but unfortunately they can also be very unreliable. News teams will cancel 'low level' stories at the drop of the hat if something more topical comes along. You need to be very patient with them – understand that they will always go with what they think is most sensational, what will cause the greatest readership/viewing figures/listener levels. That does not mean that what you have to say is not important, or that you are not interesting, just that there are other priorities at work. Never give up, always be cheerful and understanding with them and they are more likely to come back to you.

Keep looking for the 'angle'. In other words, tell your story over and over again but in different ways that make it sound very relevant to something currently big in the news. Relate popular thought and buzzwords to your own field, make the issues clearly much broader than simply you trying to find business delivering babies privately. Read and watch other stories, work out how the writer has adapted the story to make it more topical/glamorous/sensational/tragic/humorous, or whatever, in order to reach a wider audience.

Other opportunities

You may also have other opportunities to be in the public eye in person, perhaps at a function as a guest speaker, perhaps at a careers talk at a college, perhaps at a charity event. These are always worthwhile, if you have the time and are usually fun. They can always broaden awareness of your services.

Summary

- You should now understand how to recognize PR opportunities.
- Make the most of these according to your available time and confidence.
- Support any group efforts.

Advertising your services

Where to advertise

The obvious place is your local newspaper, but others include local phone directories, parish magazines, school/college newspapers and theatre programmes. You can probably think of more places than these where you have seen local businesses advertise. Then there are the expensive ones; local radio, local television, national magazines or newspapers – well, you never know, someone might sponsor you! You could have a signwriter do a beautiful job on the sides and back of the car, you can advertise in panels in the back of a taxi; there are numerous places to put an ad.

The question is, where is the most appropriate place for your advertisement, which will be costing you a large chunk of your marketing budget. Where will more of the most relevant people see it, notice it and subsequently take the trouble to contact you? This is never an easy problem for a previously unadvertised service; but you will be able to make a very good judgement based on all of the market knowledge you have now acquired, assuming you have gone through most of the processes described in this chapter. It is largely common sense – a poster in the local pub is probably very unlikely to raise any business enquiries; an ad in the local newspaper, especially if you cannot afford to run it for some weeks, is also unlikely to bring you any work. If you do decide to invest, perhaps as a group, in some form of advertising, pick something that is a one off cost, like a directory, but which will be re-used and therefore looked at many times by the consumers.

Finding information

If you wish to investigate the cost of an ad somewhere, there is a very simple process to follow. In your local library, there will be a copy of the advertising agencies' bible called 'BRAD Rates and Data'. It is a huge volume, published monthly and it is full of the 'Rate Card' information on all media that take advertising. They are listed by geographical or business area and you will be able to find the ones that interest you, copy down the phone number, then call them and ask for a sample copy (of a newspaper or magazine) and a 'media pack'. This will be sent to you, but avoid telling them you are an individual, call on behalf of an association of some kind.

Targeting

Remember that you do not want to hit a wide audience of the general public, you want to target women considering having children under private care at home. You will not be able to target them specifically, but by keeping them in mind, you will be able to decide the most sensible places to advertise.

Costs

The first cost you will have is your production costs; you will have to design or write your ad, then produce finished artwork or pay/persuade someone else to do this for you.

If you are considering a newspaper ad, there are always last minute deals to be had at a fraction of the cost of normal display advertising in the 'run of press', i.e. in the main part of the paper. There will be no negotiating in the Classified section.

Any of the advertising sales people you might contact will give you discounts off the 'rate card' (i.e. the published standard prices, like a 'rack rate' in a hotel) if you negotiate hard enough. Sometimes you can combine your advertisement with a piece of 'free' editorial.

Remember the smaller places to advertise, such as the parish magazine, will be much cheaper and will offer you more space on a page to yourself, rather than being swallowed up with hundreds of other ads on the same page.

Designing an effective ad

The primary functions of advertising are to raise awareness and to elicit some kind of response. It depends on the type of product as to how this is achieved; with your services, you really need to get someone to phone you or write to you for further information. Your design should therefore have this as its main focus. As people generally read very little advertising, pick a very, very small number of choice words, if possible a positive, active phrase, such as 'Having a baby at home could be a real bundle of joy...' followed by a brief summary of what you offer, 'Independent midwives can...', then the response mechanism, 'phone us for more information'.

There are whole books on this subject, but briefly, if in doubt, find some ads you think really work and copy their format but with your words/ pictures. This is called recycling and it works!

Once you have designed and written it, get a good number of people to read it and comment, preferably people who are similar to your target group. Then you will need to produce artwork; mostly newspapers will do this for you from your design work, unless it is very complicated. A parish magazine will probably not have the facilities, but artwork produced on a desktop publishing system at a local college will be adequate.

Summary

You should be able to place an effective advertisement that you can afford, that will have maximum impact and produce some kind of response.

CHAPTER SIX

Supervision

Role of the Supervisor of Midwives

The Midwives Rules and Code of Practice are quite specific about the role of the Supervisor within the Local Supervising Authority (LSA).

> 'The Supervisor of Midwives should give you support as a colleague, counsellor and adviser. This should be developed in order to promote a positive working relationship which is conducive to maintaining and improving standards of practice and care.' (UKCC, Midwife's Code of Practice, 1994)

It is very important that you understand the difference between a Supervisor and a manager. Occasionally, some Supervisors themselves are unclear, as they are not used to acting in a purely supervisory capacity. Managers act under the constraints of an employing authority. They are responsible for ensuring that contracts are fulfilled, and that obligations on both sides are met. If you are an employee, you have signed a contract which says what you will do, for how long at a time, and for how much. The contract should also spell out what will happen if you don't, or can't, meet these obligations. Managers also have wider responsibilities than to the individual. They have to ensure that other contracts are met, such as providing as many midwives per ward as are required for safe practice.

Supervisors, on the other hand, have a duty to the individual midwife, and to the general public. They must monitor practice as outlined in the Rules and Code of Practice, and monitor the practice of all midwives in their area, whether employed or independent. Your Supervisor's responsibility is to make sure that you are a safe practitioner, and that the public is protected from you if you are not. It is also her 'paramount responsibility' to make sure that you have:

> 'all the requisite relevant information to enable them (midwives) to function effectively within the statutory regulations and framework.'

'She also gives advice and guidance to midwives, their managers, the health authority, private maternity hospitals, agencies supplying midwives, and independent midwives.' (ENB 'Guidelines for Local Supervising Authorities', 1987)

In essence, the Supervisor may be a manager, and a manager may be a Supervisor, but not necessarily, and it is very important that these two roles do not become confused with each other. It is now mandatory that a Supervisor should have undergone the Supervisor's course before she takes up her post, rather than within a year of appointment. This should help to ensure that Supervisors have a good preparation in their role before they start.

Responsibilities of the Supervisor of Midwives

Your Supervisor should be a midwife who will work with you as an equal colleague. She should enable you to give your clients the best possible care. She can do this in a number of ways.

1. She can help you to decide which refresher courses/study days would be useful for you, and she can also make sure that you have details of any such events occurring locally.

2. She should support you in your efforts to base your practice on the available research, even (especially) if the research findings clash with local hospital policies.

3. She can be a most useful and helpful sounding board. The Rules say that she should be consulted on a number of issues, including equipment, notes and drugs. Her advice should be clear, helpful and based upon the Rules and Code of Practice.

4. She can help you to organize honorary contracts. These contracts will allow you to practice in a hospital when you bring in your own clients. Some hospitals issue general honorary contracts, some issue contracts for named women to be used if needed. Some may refuse to issue them to you. If your Supervisor is unable to facilitate this, then you may like to try another hospital. If this is not practical, then speak to the Regional Nursing Directorate, and see if they can influence the issue of a contract. There are no guarantees, however.

Finding a new Supervisor

In spite of all the above, you may occasionally find a Supervisor who is not as helpful, unbiased and friendly as you might hope. If it becomes clear that the Supervisor is not acting in the spirit of the Code of Practice, then you do have alternatives. First, if your attempts to reconcile the relationship fail, you should go to your link Supervisor. Every LSA has a Supervisor who fulfils this role. Explain the situation to her, and ask her to allocate you to another Supervisor. It may help if you make discreet enquiries in advance as to the sympathies of other Supervisors. If the link Supervisor refuses, or takes no action within a reasonable space of time, then go direct to the LSA. Explain to them why you are approaching them directly, and ask them to allocate you to another Supervisor. Finally, if they fail to help you, go to the midwifery professional adviser at the UKCC and enlist her help. There is no need for you to put up with substandard supervision, but, on the other hand, you do have an obligation, first of all, to try to make the relationship work.

Notifications

Of intention to practise

The Notification of Intention to Practise is an annual return to the LSA. The forms are sent to each practising midwife from the UKCC. On that form, it will be possible to indicate each area, within a given LSA, in which you will be practising. You send the completed form to the Supervisor of Health Authority 1, who will then send a copy to each of the other areas you have indicated. If you intend to practise in more than one LSA, you will need to send for an additional form, MID2. This notification should be sent to the Supervisors on or before March 31st each year.

Please note that, occasionally, an independent midwife has been told that her Notification to Practise has been 'refused' or 'not accepted'. It is not within the remit of any Supervisor or any LSA to refuse a Notification unless a) it has not been filled in properly, b) the midwife has been suspended from practice (not suspended from duty – see below 'Suspension'), or c) the midwife has been struck off the Register. A Notification is just that: it notifies the LSA that this midwife intends to practise in their area. It is not a request for permission to practise.

Of birth

It is normally the midwife who notifies the 'appropriate medical officer' of the birth of an infant within 36 hours of the birth, although the duty is laid upon the father, and any other person in attendance on the mother at the birth, or within six hours afterwards. Interestingly, the midwife has no similar responsibility to notify her Supervisor of Midwives, although most do as a matter of courtesy. You should ask your Supervisor for a stock of Birth Notification forms. You can always photocopy these as you need. You are under no obligation to enter the details on any hospital computer system, or indeed any other form of notification. Be aware that some health authorities have increasingly complex forms requiring subjective judgements to be recorded. The only legal requirement is that the child's birth is notified. The birth must be notified whether the child is live or stillborn.

Births must not only be notified, they must also be registered. Usually, it is the father or mother who does this, and it should be done within 42 days of the birth in the England and Wales, or 21 days in Scotland. If for any reason the parents do not register the birth, then the responsibility devolves upon any person present at the birth, including the midwife.

Of death

The midwife must notify the Supervisor of every stillbirth, neonatal or maternal death occurring 'when she is the midwife responsible for the delivery of care to the mother and her baby' (UKCC, 1991).

You must also be prepared to have to complete a death certificate for any stillbirths born to women in your care who are not registered with a GP. The Code of Practice states that you should only do this if you were present at the delivery, or examined the body. Whenever possible, you should state on the certificate the cause of death and the estimated duration of the pregnancy.

As far as registration of the death is concerned, this is primarily the duty of the relatives, but should they fail in this duty, it falls to any person who was present at the death. This applies to babies born after 24 weeks gestation.

Suspension from practice

Note carefully the subheading. It says 'practice' not duty. Your manager may, if she feels she has sufficient cause, suspend you from duty. Only the LSA, acting on advice from the Supervisor, can suspend you from actual practice. If a Supervisor tells you she is suspending you from practice, she is acting illegally. You can refer her to the Rules and Code of Practice, if you like.

As an independent, the threat of suspension from duty holds no fears for you. The threat of suspension from practice is a different matter. This affects your livelihood – suspension from duty means you continue to be paid, suspension from practice means you have no way of earning your living in the field of midwifery. There are two main grounds for suspension from practice.

1.   On health grounds, to prevent the spread of an infection, or if a midwife has been reported to the Health Committee of the UKCC.

2.   On grounds of alleged professional misconduct. This means that if you have been reported to the UKCC Preliminary Proceedings Committee, or the Professional Conduct Committee, you may be suspended by the LSA until 'any proceedings or investigations have been determined' (UKCC, 1991).

If an LSA decides to suspend a midwife, they have to report any suspension, and the grounds for it, to the UKCC forthwith, with a view to investigation and possible 'removal from the Register'. They also have to notify the midwife in writing of her suspension and the grounds for it. At least this means that the midwife has a chance to examine the case against her, and start planning a course of action.

Rules of evidence

If any Supervisor considers that you have case to answer, and wants to talk about that particular case, then she must warn you, at the outset of the meeting, that she intends to take what you say to the LSA with a view to implementing a suspension. If she does not do this, then she may have allowed you to incriminate yourself, and the evidence would not be admissible at any hearing into the case.

You should remember that you have only been suspended by one LSA, however. You are perfectly free to practice in another, unless you do something there which leads them to suspend you. They cannot suspend you on the grounds that you have been suspended by another LSA. You should note, however, that this may change. The UKCC will publicise any changes to the status quo.

Action plan

Let us assume that you do not feel that you are guilty of professional misconduct. (If you do, and you are, you should still prepare a statement of mitigation to be presented to the committee. This at least could help to minimize any professional consequences. It won't necessarily get you off the hook, though.) You will feel appalled, burning with a sense of distress and outrage. Your first task is to inform your clients, and help them to make alternative arrangements. Then contact the professional department of whichever professional body you are a member.

Enlisting help

Tell them the whole story, including any background information which they may need. They will help you to prepare your statements, in addition to the help you will receive from the legal bods and any other department whose advice would be useful. If at any time you believe that the help you are getting is not up to standard, go to the Head of the Department and say so. This is your future we're discussing – you need solid gold advice and wholehearted support. Get the best legal help you can from the very beginning.

Even if you have been professionally negligent, you are still entitled to the best you can get. That's why you pay your subscription after all. Take support from whoever offers it; you should be able to look to your Supervisor for professional assistance, but this is not always the case. Relations between you may be a little strained under the circumstances. You may prefer to make contact with a different Supervisor. Ask the link Supervisor for help, if she is not involved; if she is, ask the Regional Nursing Directorate for help. Talk to people about what is happening to you, especially your professional peers. Try to find yourself an additional source of income for the duration. At least you'll have some money coming in, and you won't be sitting brooding at home.

Read Chapter 2 for the procedures which are followed by the statutory bodies, and do take legal advice as soon as you can. Don't worry that if you take a solicitor into your confidence, or take a representative of the RCM to meetings with management, you will be perceived as escalating the situation. Nobody else will be troubled by such qualms. They won't hesitate to use any slip or unfortunate comment by you against you, so be warned. It is never too early to take proper professional advice.

Confidentiality

The question of confidentiality of information about clients can never be overstressed. Clients are entitled to have their privacy protected. Just because they have booked with you does not mean that you can inform all and sundry. In fact, you are under no statutory obligation to inform anybody that such and such a woman has booked your services, not her GP, nor even your Supervisor. Most midwives do inform their Supervisors of bookings out of courtesy, but it is incumbent upon the Supervisor to realize that this does not give her the right to transmit the information to anyone else. You need to be particularly careful when dealing with sensitive issues such as surrogacy, when the clients may prefer not to have anyone else but you know of the booking.

Confidentiality versus the public interest

Other issues which may make women feel especially private are subjects such as HIV or genital herpes. Unfortunately, these are the sort of matters that professionals have a right to know, in order that you can protect yourself and others from potential infection. Good practice in prevention of infection in all cases, however, should protect you. You should be prepared to either counsel the woman yourself, if you have the necessary skills, or to refer her to a counsellor to help her come to terms with the fact that what she has may affect other people, who therefore have a right to know. Many women prefer not to go public about a previous termination – sometimes even their partners don't know – so you need to tread very carefully, and again, may find that some counselling is needed.

You are not under any obligation to let a doctor know either, although you may find it oils the political wheels if a woman's GP is aware of her plans. You can only do this with her permission, and the same applies to informing any obstetric consultant. If a woman refuses to give her permission, or asks you not to phone or talk to a particular individual, including a Supervisor, then you may not do so. However, it may make you feel more comfortable if you can explain to the woman your own professional feelings. There may be another Supervisor that she is happy for you to talk to, especially if you are concerned about a particular aspect of her care. This aspect of professional responsibility versus the duty of confidentiality is an extremely difficult one. If you are seriously concerned, then do talk to one of the professional, or industrial relations officers, at the RCM, without giving any identifiable details, and ask for her advice. In an emergency, or if the client is not capable of giving consent (if for example, she is unconscious), then you must take the action you deem most appropriate under the circumstances. You may say that action taken is in the public interest.

You also need to guard against gossiping! When you have a batch of clients due about the same time, they love to hear what's happening to the others. However, you have to be circumspect about the level of information that you give. Many of us teach classes or clients by using anecdotes – make sure that the subject of the story is not readily identifiable. Mothers of triplets, for example, can usually be fairly accurately identified in small communities. By all means tell people that so-and-so has had her baby, and all is well, but anything else is really erring into personal information that so-and-so may not want other people to know. As far as professional colleagues such as Supervisors are concerned, it may help you to devise a form of labour summary which will give the basic information without the personal details.

One final comment. As the Royal Family has found to its cost, conversations on mobile telephones can be overhead by just about any idiot with the right equipment. If you need to have conversations on sensitive issues, do it on a land line. Any idiot needs permission from the Home Secretary to overhear these.

Summary

- Be aware of the role and responsibilities of the Supervisor of Midwives.
- Ensure your notification are up to date in all areas when you intend to practise.
- Ensure that you are a paid up member of a professional organization.
- Be aware of the legal processes involved in suspension from practice.
- Make sure that you have thoroughly considered issues of confidentiality.

CHAPTER SEVEN

Matters of Practice

Devising notes

As explained in Chapter 2, the notes must follow a format approved by the Local Supervising Authority. The information must be clearly set out, and it is useful to have a logical progression. Examples of note format can be found at the back of this book, and also in Mary Cronk and Caroline Flint's book *Community Midwifery – A Practical Guide*.

Only put in your notes the information you need. They don't need to be cluttered up with the extraneous dribs and drabs that you often find in hospital notes. If you decide to put your notes in exercise books, use good quality hardbound books. In the paper covered ones, the paper quality will deteriorate quickly. A word processor is worth its weight in gold because then you can alter and change the layout as much as you like. It also means that you don't have to have large quantities of photocopied sheets lying around; you can just print off a copy as you need it. A decent printer helps too. If you don't have a word processor, then type up a master copy of your notes, and photocopy a number of them. When you are down to your last two copies, you can print up some more. Make sure the paper is fairly resilient, as it has to last a long time. 90 gm weight paper and upwards is the best. Keep the notes inside folders, as this keeps them clean. Plastic or cardboard are best, and an opaque finish will keep them hidden from nosy glances.

Personalizing the format

Start by jotting down what you need to know on the first page – name, address, phone number etc, and then move logically through antenatal, labour and postnatal sections. The extra bits you want to put in as an independent midwife are very much up to you. You will need, however, a space for the financial arrangements, and a space for you and the client to sign the contract of agreement between you. Usually these signatures are added to the financial arrangements, so that everybody is clear. You will also need to enclose, in your copy of the notes, correspondence about this client.

Leave lots of space, particularly in your antenatal and postnatal visits section. For the labour, it may be useful to design yourself a partogram. There will certainly be bits of a hospital partogram that are of no relevance to you at all, but having things in a graph format does help to fill them in quickly, and you can allow space for your text which might include the positions the client is using, or how she was feeling at any particular time. There is an example in Appendix 3.

You should aim to make your notes comprehensive, but concise. You may also like to leave space for your client to write her own contributions. She may like to write a birth plan in case you should be unavailable for whatever reason when she goes into labour, and she has to have a substitute midwife. Document everything as it happens, and you won't get caught on the hop.

Facilitating audit of practice

Auditing your practice is a most useful exercise. Try to devise your notes in a form which will make practice audit easy. Keep details of such subjects as outcomes of alternative practices, use of different labour positions, or blood loss, for example, and make it easy to correlate these data. This is good practice for a group of midwives working together as well, as you can then look at the practice results as well as individual audit.

Booking clients – or how not to tout for trade

Preliminary visits

Booking clients assumes that you have already made a preliminary visit, and that terms and conditions have been discussed. If not, then you will need to do it at booking, and this can make the whole session a marathon effort. The preliminary visit should take place on the assumption that the woman is interested in having an independent midwife at her birth, and that you are there to see if this would be right for all concerned.

Criteria for booking

The important issues are:

1. Safety
    Does this woman want a homebirth, and is it a safe option for her and her baby? Does anything in her past history suggest that she would be better off in hospital? Does she know the limitations of the midwife's role, or does she assume that having booked you, everything will magically go according to plan? If homebirth does not seem to you to be a safe option, can you arrange something else for her? A domino may well be a good compromise.

2.   Compatibility
Does this woman feel comfortable with you? Do you feel comfortable
with her? Don't be blinded by your own pity if she tells you a
horror story of her past experiences. It may well be you that she
blames this time if things don't go her way. Do you remind her of a
girl at school that she hated? Don't be embarrassed to recommend
another midwife if it seems appropriate. What does she want from
you? It may be that she has a need for someone to depend on that
makes you uncomfortable. Do listen to your instincts, and take note
of your first impressions. If you feel uncomfortable, then you don't
have to book her. It's easier at the beginning to refuse the booking
for whatever reason than it is to try and undo the booking at a later
date. If in doubt – don't do it.

3.   Practicality
How far away does this woman live? Is it practical to book her if
she lives fifty miles on a notoriously congested road? Is there anybody
closer who could do it? Of course, if you love each other on sight,
you may be prepared to go and stay with her, or she may be able to
stay close to your home. However, it should be said that there are
two aspects to this problem. One is, how would you defend yourself
to a Supervisor if it took you two hours to get to your client and
when you did, something was dreadfully wrong; the other is that
you need to consider just what a pain the postnatal visits are going
to be, under these circumstances.

In addition, the question of practicality includes how many other
women you have booked, who are due about the same time. If you
are practising singlehanded then you really ought to think very
carefully before you book more than two women a month, and
also think how far away they are from each other. You could be
spending a very boring and tiring time on the road! Group practices,
or partnerships, can afford to be more flexible in their bookings.

4.   Cost
Can this woman afford your services, and if she can't, what are you
going to do about it? Can you afford to offer yet another 100 per
cent discount, or can you ask her what she can afford, and then
charge her that? In making these decisions, it is always helpful to
see the woman in her own home. You must also remember that if
she decides to sell her car to pay for your service, this will make
you feel awful. Grant her the courtesy of respecting her decision.
She has made this choice, to pay you by this means, and it is churlish
not to accept it with a good grace – it demonstrates just how much
she values your service. It is also none of your business. It's a good
idea to establish how much deposit should be paid, and ask to be

paid this at the booking visit. It should be a reasonable proportion of the total sum, say 25 per cent.

After the preliminary visit, it's a good idea to leave the decision for a couple of days or so to give your client and her family time to discuss the matter between themselves. You may like to point out to her that you will make note of her due date in your diary, and so would appreciate hearing from her so that you can either confirm it or rub it out. She may prefer to phone; if she doesn't want, or can't afford your service it may be easier to say no if she's not directly in your presence. If you haven't heard after a week, then ring her. You could have someone wanting to book you definitely who is due at the same time, so you can't afford to be left waiting for an answer.

Booking

The booking visit will take anything up to two hours, so make sure that you allow for this. In the hospital, or even for a community midwife, time is at a premium. You are always aware of all the other women waiting to see you for various reasons, so you try to get things done as quickly as possible. You're an independent midwife now – you can afford the time.

At this meeting you are going to ask a lot of personal questions – make sure both, or all of you are comfortable and at your ease. Some midwives feel that, if there is a possibility that the woman may have matters to discuss which even her family may not know about, they prefer to have this visit with the woman on her own. In the hospital setting, it is more usual for the woman to attend on her own, and she can be given what is often an 'edited' set of notes. In independent practice, partners and families do tend to be much more involved, so you need to be aware of the need for privacy.

There are lots of questions that require a simple 'yes' or 'no' answer, but there are a great many more which need amplification. Try to ask open ended questions, and do vary the routine in which you ask them. This keeps you alert for odd bits of information, or attitudes which may help you and your client plan her care more effectively. Use this time to begin a preliminary plan for her care and for the birth, by assessing those things which are important to her. Encourage her to talk about her hopes and fears; find out what she wants from you; talk about her past experiences. You must be realistic – there may be areas of experience, such as delivering breech babies, about which you feel less confident. You must be honest. You won't be diminished in anyone's eyes if you're frank about the limits of the care you are able, realistically, to offer. Do consider between you what will happen if she needs to be transferred in. Most independents are able to arrange honorary contracts with their clients' local hospitals to stay with their clients and deliver the baby if possible. If this client's local hospital is unhelpful in this respect, then ask another one if they would be able to help if a transfer, or advice were required.

Once you've finished completing the information you both need, you do an antenatal examination, and you're finished. One of the exciting things about carrying a sonicaid (or similar) is that you can hear the fetal heart really early, sometimes from about ten weeks, and, more to the point, so can the woman. This moment of great joy she may well want to share with her partner and any other children. Children, even quite little ones, often feel that this is what makes the baby real for them, and remember that moment well after the birth of their new brother or sister.

Late bookings

You may well find that women book you at very different stages in their pregnancy. It's always nice to get an early booking – it gives you and your client a chance to make a very close bond. However all independent midwives at some point get a desperate call from a woman in very late pregnancy (one woman even rang an independent midwife to come to her when she was in labour, so disenchanted was she with her allocated midwife!). You may have to do a very hasty booking that same day, or the next. You may find yourself having to notify your intention to practice after the event, so don't forget to contact the local Supervisor personally, and explain the circumstances. It is not a statutory requirement, but it is a professional attitude, and will facilitate future relationships in the area.

Confidentiality

Do try not to involve yourself in any dispute between the local midwives and your client. Unless you feel that the service has been so bad that the midwives in question need counselling from their Supervisor, you could find yourself in deep water if you don't know all the relevant facts. You should also remember that the client may not wish you to discuss her case with anyone else, so ask for her consent before you talk to the Supervisor. If she feels that the Supervisor is in some way involved with what has happened to her, then ask your client before writing a brief but courteous note to say you have been, or are, involved in the care of this client, which may serve the purpose (see the section on 'Confidentiality' for a deeper exploration of this problem).

Caring for women with special needs

Women with special needs may present you with a need to seek advice. Travellers and Romany families often fare badly at the hands of the established service. In some areas, there are community midwives with a particular interest in working with these women, but they are few and far between. Also, the liaison between different areas often fails to provide a continuity of care which may benefit women who live on the road. At least if they are booked with an independent midwife, you can make it your business to liaise with another practitioner of their choice, if they are not going to actually give birth with you. You need to ensure that they have all the basic work done, and give them some notes to carry wherever they go. They are entitled to the ordinary facilities, such as blood tests and scans if they want them, and you can organize these, through your Supervisor if necessary.

If you book a woman who is disabled, be very sure that you are going to be able to fulfil, or at least facilitate the fulfilment of, her particular needs. Find out from her how you can best help her, and then go and ask advice from appropriate sources. Deaf women, for example, may be able to lipread well, but only if you are facing them, with your face in a reasonable light, and speaking normally. Talking slowly and carefully distorts normal speech patterns and renders you incomprehensible. If she uses sign language as her normal means of communication, then you need a competent signer to interpret. Blind women may like to have a braille copy of their notes – how can you do this, and ensure confidentiality is maintained? If she wants to deliver in hospital, can you organize a room for her which will not be full of traps and pitfalls? Can she have repeated visits to the ward to familiarize herself, or would it be better to plan on a domino, so that she can come home early? Will wheelchair-bound women be able to get about in the hospital, or does it seem likely that narrow doorways and cluttered spaces will prevent her? Would she also be better with a domino delivery or a homebirth, so that she can be in her own accustomed space as soon as possible? How could these options be facilitated, and are they practical? A disability does not mean that options are limited – it simply means that you have to be creative in your thinking and planning. It also means that if you think you are not going to be able to help this woman, you should not book her. She is likely to require very specialist input at some point or another – are you the right person to supply this, or could someone else do it better? Be honest with yourself and with her, and don't let your desire to help get the better of your common sense.

'Transferring in'

The important thing about transferring to consultant care is to accept that there will be occasions when it is the only sensible thing to do. Don't look on transfer, as some midwives and their clients do, as some sort of failure. It isn't. It's the responsible action of a trained professional who understands the limits of her expertise. Sometimes you feel that when you get there the hospital midwives will sneer at you, and imply that they knew you would need them in the end – especially if you have booked someone whose care has not been that straightforward. In practice, this attitude is very rarely evident, and you will quickly earn respect for transferring appropriately, rather than battling on for too long at home with dicey results.

Antenatal transfers

If your client needs to transfer in pregnancy, this is usually due to some condition caused by the pregnancy, which will require specialist obstetric assistance to maintain a successful pregnancy, or at delivery. This may apply to women who develop insulin dependent diabetes for example, or who are found to have placenta praevia. You may perhaps diagnose twins; unless you are very experienced and have a midwife partner, or have a colleague who is, and who would be prepared to act as responsible midwife, you would be dangerously unwise to even contemplate homebirth.

Personal practice limits

There are grey areas: how long after rupture of membranes do you suggest that induction may be a reasonable option? After 12 hours? 24? After you've exhausted all the other methods of 'natural' induction? What is your cut off point, in terms of gestation, before which you would not like your client to deliver at home? At what point do you decide to stay with the woman, rather than going at intervals to see how she is progressing with her early labour? You need to know, to have worked these out, before the situation ever arises. Now that you no longer have to abide by hospital policies, your own professional guidelines have to be properly considered with regard to the available research.

Emotional needs

Do be aware that if you need to transfer in to hospital, your client may well perceive this as a reflection on her personal capability; the 'Couldn't even get this right' syndrome. It is your responsibility to help her to realize that this is not a failure in anybody's terms, except, perhaps, her own. She needs to know that these things happen in labour, and that it is not a 'fault' in her, just the luck of the draw. She is more likely to take it badly if she feels bulldozed into a decision. If you both arrive at this conclusion together, and after you have taken her through what is happening, she is more likely to view transfer positively. This does imply, however, that you have time to do all this. Sometimes you need to act quickly. One tip is to use the words 'we' or 'us' when advising of the need to transfer urgently, for example, 'The baby isn't responding very well to the labour, and his heartbeat is rather slow. We need to ask an obstetrician for his help, so it would be better if we went to the hospital'. Yes, it's a bit gooey, but you're making it clear that you're in this together, and that you're not going to desert her.

Communicating effectively

Occasionally, you'll be faced with what is effectively a refusal from the woman to go to hospital when you would infinitely prefer that she did. Be as persuasive as you can, and explain to her and her partner why this move is best. If she won't transfer, try to understand why. If the move is urgently needed, then don't worry about letting her see your anxiety. If you stay icy cool, she may not pick up your sense of urgency. I'm not saying that you should heap ashes on your head and tear your clothing, but use your own strong feelings as a woman and as a professional (if any male midwives are reading this, I'm assuming that your empathy levels are pretty high, too!).

If the mother refuses to leave her home, despite your advice, you should document this, and continue to provide care. Try to contact your Supervisor as well; her support can be invaluable in this situation. You will need to contact her at some point to inform her of the woman's refusal to transfer, and the sooner the better. It is always more traumatic to transfer in second stage. If you suspect that transfer may be needed, it is better to discuss transfer earlier rather than later.

One midwife faced with this situation rang her Supervisor to inform her of the event. Minutes later, the doorbell rang, and there was the Supervisor on the doorstep. It soon became clear that the Supervisor had arrived to help and support the midwife in caring for the woman. Later, when the woman herself had finally suggested that transfer would be a good idea, the Supervisor followed the ambulance in her car, and waited until an overdue caesarean section had been performed. Then she made the midwife some tea, and took her back to the client's house, where she helped to clear up. This, the midwife felt, was not so much supervision as sainthood.

Transfer during labour

Transfer in labour usually presents as one of two scenarios. Either your client is getting nowhere very slowly, and both of you need some help, or you need to transfer fast as some emergency is looming. With slow progress, it is important to differentiate between a long pre-labour stage, and actual failure to progress in terms of cervical dilatation and descent of the presenting part. Your client may need an epidural because she is exhausted, in great pain, and the baby is still in occipito-posterior position. You will have time to do all the things that need to be done, such as pack her a bag and see about childcare, so that her partner can come too, instead of having to stay with the children.

Some midwives transfer clients when they notice meconium stained liquor, and some don't. Some transfer if the meconium staining looks fresh, and not if it appears, in their clinical judgement, to be due to postmaturity. If you are happy to stay home with a baby who has meconium stained liquor, you must have good suction equipment, and may like to have a second midwife present.

Dealing with emergencies

There are very few things that happen in midwifery which require that you transfer the woman ten minutes ago, but if it does look like that, don't panic. Remember, your client and her partner are probably more frightened than you are, so your first responsibility is to maintain an atmosphere of calm competence. Tell them exactly what is happening, and explain that you need to transfer to the hospital, and what they can expect when they get there. Do be concise.

Calling for help

Call an ambulance, or the flying squad. Some people think that clients of independent midwives are not entitled to the flying squad, but this is a myth. If you call an ambulance, tell them who you are, and what help you need. If you have a woman who has just had an eclamptic fit, it's no good having ambulance personnel rushing noisily into the house expecting to help at an emergency delivery. You need experienced paramedics if you live in an area with no flying squad. Many areas, if not most, have now abandoned flying squads as they take personnel away from where they are most needed. Stress to ambulance control that you need paramedic assistance, and why, when you call them. After that call, phone the obstetric team, and speak to the senior registrar, or the registrar. With the best will in the world, the houseman may be no use at all, being probably less experienced than you are.

Do the observations and procedures you have been trained to do in this type of emergency, and jot down the timings of the calls you have just made, and to whom they were made. If you are having to concentrate on your client or her baby, ask the partner to quickly note these down. If the house is difficult to find, ask the partner to wait at a convenient spot close to the house to indicate its whereabouts. This assumes that you are on your own, and there is no lonelier time in all the world than this. Many independents prefer to work in pairs at a delivery, but it isn't always possible.

Emergency procedures

If you think an intravenous infusion is likely to be needed – especially if the woman is haemorrhaging – then put one up. You will, of course, be carrying the appropriate solutions; anaesthetists recommend that you use Hartmanns Solution in the first instance, and that a litre should be sufficient until help arrives. The ambulance should carry Gelufusin or Haemaccel, but you would be well advised to have this ready in case it is needed. *Don't put an intravenous infusion into a baby* unless you have been trained to do this, have had plenty of practice, know it is needed and are confident.

Your observations and recordings should be red hot – you may be certain that if they're not, someone will notice, and you'll find yourself on the proverbial carpet. As independents, our practice is often more closely observed than other midwives, and you need to be spotless as far as records are concerned.

Debriefing

If there have been two of you involved, get together as soon as you can and talk about it. You both need to unload, and to confirm with each other emotionally that you did your best. If you have been on your own, then find someone to share it with. Almost certainly it will be most useful to talk about it with another midwife. Your life partner, if not a midwife, will not understand the finer points, and although sympathetic, will not be able to make the judgements you need. A sympathetic Supervisor is probably the best of all possible options.

You should be prepared, whatever the outcome, to discuss it with the Supervisor, and possibly, at a perinatal mortality meeting. This can be distressing, so take a companion with you, if you feel you need that support. If two of you were present, then go to any meeting together, and make sure that your notes will bear the level of intensive scrutiny they are likely to get.

Research

Applying it to practice

As stated earlier, many hospital policies seem to have no basis in currently available research. To consider an example, let's take routine artificial rupture of membranes. In the absence of supporting evidence, the World Health Organization still maintains that routine artificial rupture of membranes is a practice that should be stopped. There is no evidence to suggest that in a normal pregnancy and labour this practice is useful, in that it deprives the fetus of the protection of the amniotic sac, and increases the strength of contractions without measurable benefit, especially in first labours. The available research does not back the practice, but it is routinely performed, without apparent question, all over the country.

You may sometimes find yourself in a situation which requires you to defend your practice. You must be able to justify your action (or inaction) convincingly. The best way to do this is to point to the available research to support your judgement. Obviously, you can't do that if the research isn't there! Use the *Guide to Effective Care in Pregnancy and Childbirth* (Enkin, Keirse and Chalmers, 1995) as a bible in these circumstances, and read the section on 'Forms of care that should be abandoned in the light of the available evidence' – it makes illuminating reading.

There are many groups for those with an interest in research generally, or in a specific area. If you have a particular interest, there is usually a society, or a self help group, on that subject – sometimes both – where you can obtain up to the minute information. Pre-eclampsia is an example, or Sudden Infant Death Syndrome. If you can't find an existing group, then start one. After all, if you're interested, there are bound to be others with whom you can pool knowledge. Write letters to known experts in your field of interest, and to professional journals asking for information. Subscribe to MIDIRS and do data searches. You will probably find fifteen others areas which look fascinating as well!

You may also like to be involved in research of your own in addition to your practice audit. Areas currently of interest include whether to suture perineal tears or not; perineal massage in labour; positions for breech delivery; number and timing of antenatal visits. These should be enough to get you thinking of aspects of care which particularly interest you. Before you begin your research, enlist the help of someone experienced in the field, so that you set it up properly from the outset.

Evaluation

One of the definitions of a profession is that it uses research to further its practice. Midwives are not always as good as they might be about using research findings to influence how they do what they do, and to whom. This doesn't mean that you slavishly follow every finding which makes its way into the professional press. It means that you learn to evaluate research findings, to assess the methodology, and, in general, if it looks like a worthwhile and well structured effort, how you can incorporate it into your practice. Personal prejudice has no place in proper evaluation. You have to put any bias to one side and assess the work on its merits.

Assess methodology rigorously. If reading research is new to you, then read the first chapter in *Effective Care in Pregnancy and Childbirth*. This tells you how research studies are devised, and how biases are excluded. You should also read the three volumes entitled *Midwifery Practice* on ante, intra and postnatal care (Alexander, 1990). These books are well written, explanatory of the issues involved, and an enormous help in formulating bases for your own practice. Other reading is listed in the references at the back of the book.

Summary

- Plan your notes, and get the format approved by the Supervisor, with a view to auditing practice.
- Assess your potential clients carefully, and allow time for decisions to be made.
- Prepare ground for transfer and emergencies before you take on clients.
- Talk to Supervisors and doctors.
- Read research avidly, and base your practice upon sound models.

CHAPTER EIGHT

Smoothing the Way

Interfacing with other professionals

All through this book are references to our fellow professionals – midwives, obstetricians, GPs. You can add to the list paediatricians and health visitors. There may well be others, but these are the professionals you are most likely to be dealing with. Do not assume that you are likely to be welcomed with open arms by all these people, but do bear in mind that if you show professionalism in your attitudes and judgement, you will eventually be accepted as someone who is an expert in her field. You don't need to be friends with the whole world.

Health professionals

Working with doctors

Obstetricians and GPs sometimes find the very existence of independent midwifery a difficult concept to grasp. Our sureness that pregnancy and birth are essentially normal events, unless or until proven otherwise is anathema to people who believe in the pathological nature of childbearing. Be patient, and don't try to evangelize unless you think it will be useful. Do appreciate those doctors who support what you are trying to do. They are worth their collective weight in gold. There are not many of them, and they too come under pressure to fall into line.

It is sometimes disturbing for some doctors to realize that you are outside their sphere of control; that you don't have to follow their policies, that you have diagnostic skills, and that they cannot alter how you practise. For those doctors who think of midwives as nurses, this display of independence cuts at the heart of their power base, which may make for tricky relationships. You can't alter this mode of thinking just by talking or by being nice. It is your very existence which is the irritant. You just have to make sure that your practice will bear all the scrutiny that can be brought to bear upon it, and that your professionalism is beyond reproach. Sooner or later, they'll get used to you, but it may be difficult at times. Take comfort and support from your fellow independents, and be happy in the knowledge that it's attitudes like these that women are beginning to reject.

It always helps if you keep people appropriately informed. This does not mean you have to tell everyone who claims to have an interest in your client exactly what is happening with her (see 'Confidentiality'). Your client's GP, if he or she wishes to remain involved, would almost certainly appreciate a letter from you saying that your client has booked you, and asking what involvement with the care/labour/delivery the GP would like.

It may be helpful to include a short spiel informing the GP of the legal position; often GPs think that although you may have booked the woman, they still retain some legal responsibility. In your letter, assure them that the responsibility for your practice is yours alone, as an autonomous practitioner, and that the GP is free to offer as much or as little care as they wish. Tell them that if they do not wish to be involved with a homebirth, this is not a problem as you have direct rights of referral to obstetricians. You can also reassure them that you will keep them informed of her progress. On the other hand, if they are keen to be part of the woman's care, welcome their assistance and support, and ask them if they would like to be present at the delivery, or if they would simply like to be kept posted of events.

Working with midwife colleagues

Other midwives tend to overlap in certain specific areas. It may be that your client has booked you for the birth, and is having her community midwife do the ante and postnatal care. Under those circumstances, you will naturally want to do some antenatal visits, although these may be few in number. Liaise with the community midwife, and work out with her and the client when you will do the antenatal visits. This will save her having to repeat your work. You could document your findings in the co-op card as well as your notes, which will show that the care has been done. If your client has asked you to attend her birth because, for example, her midwife is not experienced at waterbirths, you could ask the client if her midwife could also attend. This may help to boost the midwife's confidence as well as increasing her competence.

Hospital midwives will almost certainly have heard about you, even if they have never met you before. Attitudes tend to vary. Always expect a courteous and helpful welcome, but be prepared for some midwives who may feel that what you are doing is unsafe. Unless you have been invited to give a talk, don't be tempted to embark on a justification of your practice. This is not the time, and it probably won't help. If you are referring a client, always be specific about who you want to see. If you know perfectly well that all this woman needs is half an hour on the monitor, try to arrange it with the, midwife on the phone in advance. Don't just turn up. If you are transferring a woman in labour who needs a caesarian section pronto, then talk to an obstetrician. You don't need the labour ward sister's permission first. Once people get to know you, they will accept that you know what you're talking about.

Inter-midwife contracts

If you are likely to need support from another independent midwife, then do try to arrange this cover in good time. You should make absolutely clear, between you, that you both understand exactly what is being asked, and how much is being offered. Money, that is. These, after all, are inter-midwife contracts. You are asking a professional to do work on your behalf, and a fee is due for that. If you are asking her to be on call for a client, in case you are away, offer her an on-call fee. She may not accept that, and say that you will only be liable to pay a fee if she is actually called, but in any case you are asking her to set aside time on your behalf. If there is time, write to each other, confirming what has been discussed, and documenting any payment arrangements. That way there is no room for misunderstanding.

If you are ill, or with another client and urgently need cover, there may not be time for an exchange of letters. In this case, sort out clearly on the phone just what percentage of the fee will be paid to the other midwife, and when you intend to resume care, if that is your intention. If this sounds rather formal, it's meant to. Our relationships with each other are far too important to jeopardize over ill-considered and ad hoc arrangements. Trust is important, but we're talking professional contracts here!

Seeking medical assistance

As far as doctors are concerned, you are not now an employee of an institution, with all the hierarchical implications that that involves. You are a practising, and equal, professional, with a duty to exercise your judgement in your client's best interests. As an autonomous practitioner, you have to advise your client to the best of your ability. If that means asking a doctor for a professional opinion, do it. Don't think that, even though an abnormality has occurred, you've dealt with it successfully before and you can now. Rule 40 is quite specific; you must seek medical assistance in the event of an abnormality being diagnosed. This may take the form of simply informing a doctor of a certain situation, or you may feel that it would be more appropriate for your client to see an obstetrician or a GP. In any case, you advise your client of your opinion. She may not take your advice, but that's her privilege. Tell your Supervisor, and you have done your duty under the Rules.

If you and your client decide to seek advice from a doctor, try to make sure that he has the relevant information, in writing. Your client could take a letter, along with her copy of the notes, and you could accompany her if she would like this. Arrange the visit in advance, either directly with the doctor concerned, or with whoever organizes his consultations. It is sometimes useful to speak directly with the doctor. If you know that one obstetrician is more likely to be sympathetic than another, then refer your client to the former. You don't have any obligation to any particular doctor – your obligation is to make sure that your client gets the sort of advice which is most in accordance with her needs.

Arranging the 'baby check'

As a general rule, babies are examined, at some point after the birth, by a doctor, although there is no statutory obligation to do this. Some midwives consider that a baby only requires seeing by a doctor if there appears to be a problem. In most cases, this would be a GP, or, in hospital, a member of the paediatric team. There may be instances where the woman does not want her GP to do this examination, or is not registered with a GP, and may ask you to arrange for her to see a paediatrician. Many paediatricians do work privately, and it is easy for you to ask one to come to the woman's home to do a routine baby check if she wishes. Some midwives have contact with a paediatrician whose opinion they particularly respect, and in addition to baby checks, may refer directly if a baby appears to have a problem.

Handing over to the health visitor

Health visitors can be a source of enormous help and support to new mothers. They have access to information on numerous issues of relevance and importance to the family. If the relationship is good, then the woman will have a friend and supporter for many years; at least until the present child starts school. Occasionally, the woman may be uncomfortable with the advice she has received from her health visitor, and solicit your advice. Weighing the baby can sometimes be a fraught procedure if the health visitor does not think the baby is gaining weight on a regular basis. It is important that you make yourself aware of the normal weight gain patterns in breast and bottle fed babies so that, should you be asked, you are in a position to give the woman accurate advice. If the health visitor is right to be concerned, you can help the woman to improve the situation with your expertise in this field. If not, it may be helpful to make an appointment to see the health visitor, and explain that your client is confused by the advice she has been given. You might then discuss with the health visitor why she is worried about this baby, and see if there is anything you can do, particularly information sharing, that will help. It may be useful to take relevant data references with you, so that the health visitor can check them herself at her leisure.

Clients' relatives

You may find that although the woman herself may be quite happy with her choice of place and care for the birth, her relatives may have a degree of anxiety. For fathers, this is often quite difficult, as they may truly believe that their partner is risking the baby's life by not having it in hospital. It is important to remember that fathers sometimes do have a sense of impotence during pregnancy, in that they may feel themselves relegated to the sidelines. This sensation of uselessness may lead to them being fairly assertive over decisions over which they can have influence – such as the place of birth. If you understand their feelings, you can help the couple to discuss, effectively, any differences between them. In these discussions, you can also help to air hopes and fears, aspirations and trepidations, so that by the end of the pregnancy both parties feel they have contributed to the final plan of care.

Helping partners in their role

It is also useful for partners, particularly first timers, to attend antenatal classes together. This is not always easy, as most NHS classes tend to be held in the daytime, when pregnant women have either finished work, or are allowed, under the regulations governing maternity care, time off. However, local branches of the National Childbirth Trust (NCT) hold classes which are almost always in the evening, and intended particularly for couples. These will help fathers to share the experience with others in the same boat, and to learn how to make the most of their role. Although these classes are paid for by the individuals concerned, there are facilities for reductions and even waiving of class fees for those on low incomes.

Other relations may also feel the need to load the pregnant woman with their fears and prejudices. It may help if you take up your traditional role as advocate for the woman, if you feel she has had enough at any point, and undertake to discuss concerns with the relation in question. It would also help your client to be in touch with other women who have made the same choices as she has. The local Homebirth Support group can be very useful, as can Association for Improvements in Maternity Services (AIMS) and the NCT. Both these latter groups have branches in almost every area of the country.

Running support groups

If you live in an area where there is little support of this nature, you could try running a drop-in group for your clients past and present, with a standing invitation to any other woman who would like to come to talk about her options. You may only start off with one or two women, but as the word spreads, you'll find that the numbers pick up to respectable levels. This may take a little while though, so don't expect your group's membership to rise to double figures for a few months. Running groups like this is good publicity for you anyway, and it does give women a forum for discussing issues surrounding their pregnancies. You don't have to have a fixed plan, just let the women talk about what they want at each meeting – you'll be there to answer specific points, to keep the ball rolling and to make yourself available. You may, if you're feeling ambitious, branch out to teaching antenatal classes yourself. These could be run as active birth classes (à la Janet Balaskas), antenatal swimming classes, or stretch classes – anything, in fact, which gathers groups of pregnant women together to gain support and strength from each other.

Setting your own limits

As an independent practitioner, you are responsible for deciding which women you are happy booking. Listen to your instincts. You may feel uncomfortable with a woman for no apparent reason at all, but if you feel unhappy, you don't have to book her. As an independent, you do have that final sanction. It seems brusque, to say the least, to say to someone, 'I'm sorry, but I just don't feel comfortable with you'. Most people aim to have some time after the preliminary meeting before formally booking the woman. You may find it kinder to say, perhaps, that you have been looking at your diary, and you're rather worried about the number of clients you have due at the same time as this woman. You may find that she felt the same about you, and that she decides not to book with you anyway. Some midwives have a policy of never booking people who haggle about money, or who complain about the amount. (This is different, of course, from people who explain sadly that they can't afford it. You may well feel happy about entering into negotiation with these women.)

You also have to decide the limits of your practice. Are you happy for your client with a breech baby to deliver at home with you? How many breech births have you assisted? Do you have a regular partner, or would you expect to do this alone? Would this be defensible if a tragedy occurred? How many weeks early would you be happy to attend a homebirth? Three weeks early? Four? Five? What about babies who are small for their apparent gestation? You need to be sure in your own mind a) about what feels right for you and b) what is good, safe practice.

Organizing time off

It will be important at times for you to spend time with your own family, or friends, or just for yourself. How are you going to organize this – will you ask another midwife to cover for you at pre-set times, will you work with a partner, will you take a set month off each year? Plan this in advance. Being on call 24 hours a day, every day, is crippling. Ask any midwife who has ever practised singlehanded.

In setting your own limits, you must, over the course of time, communicate these limits to your clients. It's not helpful to sit there at a first meeting, telling her what you won't do – this is intended to be a facilitating session!

How to say no

This is one of the most useful things we ever learn to do. It's rather a shame that saying 'No' gets trained out of us as children. We only have to re-learn it as adults. However, there are ways and means of saying no, and often it is easier to soften the blow with a little white lie, as discussed above.

Facing difficult case decisions

There are times when you simply have to recognize that there are limitations to an independent midwife's role. Think about the following potential clients:

1.   An insulin dependent diabetic, in her first pregnancy.

2.   A woman with a psychiatric history of paranoid schizophrenia, expecting her second baby. She had an acute psychotic episode after the first, and needed to be hospitalized for two months.

3.   A woman in her first pregnancy, with a history of renal disease, including an episode of acute kidney failure. She is currently receiving treatment for cystitis.

4.   A couple who, although they appear to have a good income, complain about the amount you are charging, and try to get you to reduce your fees. They do not say they can't afford it.

5.   A woman who wants continuity of care, but who wants an epidural and a private room, as she had with her first baby in London.

6.   A woman who had her first baby by caesarean section, because she did not make 'good enough progress' following induction of labour at term, now wants to have a homebirth.

Which of these women would you book? I have to say that the only one I would be happy with is the last. You book your clients on the basis of the use that will be made of your particular skills; four of the first five require something highly specialized, and the fifth doesn't appear to consider your skills to be of much value. Some midwives make a point of never booking anyone who hassles about the money – this is not to be confused with people who can't afford it, only those who query your worth.

Assertiveness in practice

Who else may you need to say 'no' to? What about doctors who try, or who instruct you, to perform inappropriate interventions on your client? Do you feel assertive enough to act as her advocate under these circumstances? Supervisors may try to manage you, rather than supervise you – do you feel brave enough and/or knowledgeable enough to challenge this? Practice, if necessary with aid of assertiveness classes, the art of politely, but firmly, saying no. If, in the exercise of your clinical judgement, the right thing to do is to say no, then you must be able to do it. As long as you can back it up with reference to research or the Rules and Code of Practice, you're doing fine. You don't need, or deserve, to be bullied or browbeaten. If you can demonstrate that you're right, then stick to it.

Negotiating compromises

Having said all that about feeling comfortable with saying no, learning to say 'No, but..' is also a good trick. We all have a point at which we balk; principles which we won't compromise. Some of us fight the battle for woman-centred care from the inside the NHS, some from outside, hoping to effect change through challenging the system. All of us have the same aim, however: to achieve the best in care for each individual woman, according to her individual needs. Sometimes, in order to achieve this, we have to learn the art of graceful compromise.

None of us would like to be faced with the situation that some American midwives have – they take the woman to the door of the hospital, and leave her there. We want to go with her. Once we have booked her, we want to be able to offer her our care wherever she ends up. This is the point at which you, as an independent midwife, will have to help the woman to make her decisions. If she needs to be induced, does it have to be syntocinon? Can you persuade the doctor to try prostin instead? If the Supervisor won't let you work in labour ward routinely, can you persuade her that you can care for any clients brought in as an emergency?

Negotiating to win

The art of negotiation is much the same as haggling; you need to have a price above which you will not go, and the other person has a price in mind below which they will not go. The trick is in encouraging them to believe that dropping the price has advantages in itself. For some time now, women who want to deliver in GP units, and who have reason to believe that they will not be supported by their GP in this choice, have been operating a haggling system. They go to their GP and cheerfully announce that they would like a homebirth. The GP, horrified, begs them to reconsider, and as an inducement, offers them the choice of the GP unit. The woman accepts; no face is lost, and everyone goes off happily, feeling they've won. Quite where this leaves the woman who actually wants a homebirth, I'm not sure. When the bottom line is what you want, it's difficult to start below it! I suppose they could always start negotiations by asking to deliver in the local dolphinarium.

Be that as it may, nobody ever negotiated successfully by closing off communication, so you have to start by talking to people. Try GP lunch clubs, and see if they will let you give a short talk on the advantages of, say, continuity of carer. Have plenty of documented research findings at your fingertips, and be prepared for a mixed response. Go and meet GPs and obstetricians, so that at least they know you're a reasonable human being. It may be an idea to dress to the image you're trying to put across – a tailored suit rather than jeans and sweatshirt, for example. It depends how far you're prepared to compromise your own self-image. It's interesting how many snap judgements are made on the basis of how you look.

Presenting your practice with conviction
If you are doing a presentation, perhaps to managers at your local hospital, make it as professional as you can. Have copies of papers (which you give out at the end of the meeting if possible, otherwise people will sit and read them, not hearing what you're actually saying), and carry them in neat folders. You're trying to convey the impression of a professional expert. You can't do that with crumpled pieces of handwritten paper. Again, sweet reasonableness will achieve a great deal more than anger and frustration, even if this is how you feel. Express yourself convincingly rather than forcefully. Say understanding things about other points of view, but your underlying message is that other views are mistaken. Not wrong, mistaken. Or, possibly, 'understandable in the light of how things used to be, but these days, of course, attitudes have changed/are changing' (delete where applicable).

When you find someone in a position of influence, who is receptive to your ideas, use them shamelessly. Make them feel special – they probably are. Enlist their help in changing minds or attitudes. Ask their advice, and take it. This way, you build a series of steps which will gradually achieve your goal. Be prepared to take it a step at a time, and with any luck, by the time you have achieved your goal, nobody will notice. It'll just be there, and they won't remember a time when it wasn't. If there has to be a loser, and it turns out to be you, be graceful in defeat. Minimize the damage, and hang on to your steely determination to try again later. If the loser is someone else, do be magnanimous, otherwise they'll fester away underground somewhere, and you won't see it until too late.

Summary

- Make contact with medical colleagues, accept their feelings and work, patiently, for change.
- Make opportunities to talk to other NHS midwives.
- Make formal contracts with other independent midwives.
- Facilitate relationships.
- Set your limits and learn to negotiate.

CHAPTER NINE

Expanding the Practice

Finding a partner

If you don't have a partner to start with, as soon as you get busy, you'll wish you had. Being on call all day, every day, is exhausting and demoralizing. It also means that if you want to have a holiday, you miss out on clients. If you want a week off, you can't realistically book clients for that week, or the week before, or the week after. If you want two weeks, that means six weeks altogether. So, you either arrange cover which can prove expensive, or you find a partner. This isn't always easy. There ought to be an agency, like a marriage bureau. You are looking for someone who is, in a way, as close to you as a life partner. She must think in a similar way to you, share your prejudices, and yet complement you in areas where you may lack experience, or ability, or just enjoy doing the bits you don't.

Using the grapevine

First of all, put the word out. Never underestimate the grapevine. It's effective, efficient and cheap. Ask around the local hospitals – who's rocking the boat at the moment? Are there midwives who you remember as being compatible, who perhaps can't practice at the moment because they have young children? Anyone you remember as leaving midwifery in despair at not being able to practice fully, and who is currently doing something else? Does anyone know someone who might fit the bill?

Trial periods

Once you've found someone you think will match your requirements, talk through everything you can imagine on sharing a practice. This includes money, time off, personal limitations, experience needed, confidence, attitudes towards client driven care, and all the rest. Then give it a three month trial. If, at the end of the trial period, it hasn't worked, then say goodbye. Don't think that people change once they're in a stable relationship – they don't. Slapdash or careless practice, irritating habits and control freaks will become more annoying (or more of a liability) as time progresses, not less.

If you find that there is sufficient potential business, and you are already in a successful partnership, you may need to increase your numbers further by taking on one or possibly two new members. Do all the above again, only more carefully, because there are now two people's needs to be satisfied, plus the needs of the new member(s). Personality issues are incredibly important, as the dynamics of the relationships will shift and change with new input. Some people say that threesomes are notoriously difficult to run (ask any mother of three children) and that new members should only be appointed in pairs. The theory runs that the more independent midwives there are, the greater the demand, so don't be too afraid that there won't be enough business for more independents in an area. Business may be slow for a while, but slowly and surely it will pick up as more and more women become aware of your presence and your service.

Working out back up

You may not wish to operate a partnership, but would prefer to operate as individuals offering support and back up to each other. This is fine, but it does require a certain amount of formal arrangement (see the section in Chapter 3 on 'partnerships', for contracts that you may need to organize between you). You also need to remember that without a partnership agreement, no matter how loose, other midwives' own clients take precedence, for them, over yours. This may lead to unhappy situations where you believed your client was covered by another midwife, who has had to go to a woman she has booked. There you are, out enjoying yourself, believing that all eventualities are covered, and your client has had to call an NHS midwife because you were unobtainable. Bad for business, and worse for your reputation. The moral of this is, that without a partner, you are always on call.

Tendering to health authorities

There may come a time when you perceive a niche within the existing local structure that would suit you down to the ground. A need may not be being met for women in your area; for example, waterbirths, or homebirths, may be difficult for women to achieve because of lack of local expertise. This niche could be filled by you full time, or in addition to your independent practice. Your mission, therefore, is to persuade the local purchasers that you should be offered a contract to carry out this work.

Assessing the market

First, you need to assess potential local response to your request. You are bidding for a serious contract – assuming you are practising with a partner, is the demand likely to be too much for you? Will you need extra midwives? You need to cost your services realistically. Include everything, cost of travel, midwives' hourly rates, cost of consumables – all of it. You also need to consider whether it would be more appropriate to offer a subcontracted service to the local hospital. Would they be relieved to have you take on this responsibility, or would they be unwilling? There are examples of tenders in the appendix section which you could adapt for the service you propose, but do remember that unless you have a record of competence in the area, you are unlikely to be considered as a serious provider.

Once you have put your tender together, submit it to the purchasers. The problem with informing your Supervisor of your plans is that she may well be your business rival. Don't ever give figures away without a very good reason. The local hospital may well undercut you if they know in advance what you are proposing to charge, even if they know they can't maintain the costs without cutting the service they offer to women. It will be too late by then, and your bid will have failed.

Bidding for extra contractual referrals

At the back of this book is an example of a tender to establish a Homebirth team, using independent midwives. You will, of course, need to do costings and so forth for your own particular area, but this will serve as a guide to the sort of information required for any tender. You can make a bid for any midwifery service, from taking antenatal classes through to establishing permanent premises. The type of information that you need to give stays the same, whatever the ultimate proposal.

1.   Staff involved – midwives, assistants, cleaners and so on.

2.   Roles and responsibilities.

3.   The scope of the service offered.

4.   The costs, and a breakdown of those costs.

5.   Equipment supplied, and whose responsibility is the maintenance and replacement.

This should cover all eventualities. You will need to expand each section, but don't make it too long. Concise clarity should be your watchword.

Be prepared for negotiation of the costs. They will try to get blood out of the stone. You must have in mind a figure, below which it will not be economically viable for you to go. If you get offered a tender, one last thing. Let every independent midwife in the country know about it. It will be a cause for unlimited celebration!

Opening premises

If, having read Chapter 3, you are still determined to open premises for the furtherance of your practice, then think about the possibility of opening a centre which will enable women to give birth there, and stay postnatally, rather than just using a place for antenatal consultations.

For your premises, look at the possibility of renting a part of a house, or perhaps offices in an existing health care facility (a health centre, or an alternative medicine practice). You could rent some offices, with a loo, in the town, but unless you can negotiate a low start rent, you could find these prohibitively expensive. Then read Chapter 3 again.

Funding

In order to open a centre, you will, of course, need to lay comprehensive plans. You will have to raise large amounts of money, which, given current constraints, will probably have to be raised from the private sector. Go and talk to people who are experienced in the health care field, but be selective. Try to approach those who have experience in nursing homes – they are the people who are most likely to understand your concept. Sponsorship, or fundraising, is an option, but it can be very time-consuming. Talk to local consumer or health groups about whether they would be prepared to support your project before you embark upon a major scheme. If they are supportive, then enlist their practical help in fundraising – they've probably had a lot of practice. Venture capitalists should be your last port of call – they will want everything you possess, and your soul, in addition to a life interest in your close family.

Planning

Choose what sort of facility you want to provide, and then work out how it will be economically viable. How many beds will you need to provide? How many birthing rooms will you need to service that number of beds? Will you want to provide antenatal classes? You'll need to have sufficient space for that. How many midwives will you need, and how much will you pay them? What about midwifery assistants? Will you have doctors involved? How much will insurance cost you? What about extras such as birthing pools? How will you cover emergencies?

Registration

You will need to register your premises under the Nursing Homes legislation. This means close contact with the local authority, the council and the Health Authority – possibly more than one, if you cross borders between one authority and the next. You will need to co-ordinate your efforts with the Supervisor, as she has the final say on staffing levels, and equipment needed.

You must have an idea about the ambiance of the centre you propose to establish. Is it going to be a cool, white, clinical place, or a soft, warm house, or would you consider using an existing, but unused, part of a hospital? Will you buy it, rent it or lease it? Would you convert your own house? Would your family like that? What about car parking and access – you'll need plenty of both.

Think big. The NHS won't change unless it's challenged – all monoliths need pushing at the top before they tumble, and fixed ideas in any service are about as monolithic as you can get. The more of us prepared to challenge the system from the top, the better. That way, midwives return to their position as experts in their field, and women get the care, and the choice of care they deserve. Who said changing the world was easy?

Good luck.

Summary

- If you need a partner, choose carefully and take your time over it.
- Plan and cost tenders in close detail before submitting them.
- If you decide to open premises, investigate all the aspects involved before writing your business plan, and take advice from experts.

References

Alexander, J., Levy, V., Roch, S. (1990). *Midwifery Practice.* 3 Vols. London: Macmillan.

Bond, M. (1991). *Assertiveness for Midwives.* Distance Learning Centre.

Campbell, R., MacFarlane, A. (1987). *Where to be Born – the Debate and the Evidence.* Oxford: NPEU.

Cronk, M., Flint, C. (1989). *Community Midwifery, A Practical Guide.* London: Heinemann Medical Books.

Davis, E. (1987). *Heart and Hands.* Berkeley, California: Celestial Arts.

Department of Health (1993). *Changing Childbirth. The Report of the Expert Maternity Group.* London: HMSO.

Donnison, J. (1988). *Midwives and Medical Men.* London: Historical Publications.

English National Board (1987). *Guidelines for Local Supervising Authorities.* London: ENB.

Enkin, M., Keirse, M., Chalmers, I. (1995). *A Guide to Effective Care in Pregnancy and Childbirth.* Second Edition. Oxford: Oxford University Press.

Flint, C. (1986). *Sensitive Midwifery.* Oxford: Butterworth-Heinemann.

Garcia, J., Kilpatrick, R. (1991). *The Politics of Maternity Care.* Oxford: Oxford University Press.

Golding, J., Greenwood, R., Birmingham, K. et al. (1992). 'Childhood cancers, intramuscular vitamin K and pethidine given during labour'. *British Medical Journal,* Vol. 305, No. 6849, pp. 341–46.

House of Commons Health Committee (1992). *Report on Maternity Services.* (Winterton Report). London: HMSO.

Oakley, A. (1984). *The Captured Womb.* Oxford: Blackwell.

Robinson, S., Thomson, A. (1991). *Midwives, Research and Childbirth.* London: Chapman and Hall.

Tew, M. (1990). *Safer Childbirth? A Critical History of Maternity Care.* London: Chapman and Hall.

UKCC (1985). *Advertising by Registered Nurses, Midwives and Health Visitors.* London: UKCC.

UKCC (1987). *Confidentiality.* London: UKCC.

UKCC (1991). *A Midwife's Code of Practice.* London: UKCC.

UKCC (1991). *Midwives Rules.* London: UKCC.

UKCC (1992). *Standards for Administration of Medicines.* London: UKCC.

UKCC (1993). *Standards for Records and Record Keeping.* London: UKCC.

World Health Organization (1992). *Definition of a Midwife.* Copenhagen: WHO.

What is an Independent Midwife?

Independent midwives are fully trained midwives who have chosen to work outside the NHS. As independent midwives we believe that our service is in tune with mothers' expressed wishes and needs during their pregnancy and labour. We are always happy to advise any woman on any aspect of maternity care, whether she is booked with us or not.

We offer continuity of care...

One of the most important issues to a pregnant woman is to know the midwife who will be at the birth of the baby. We promise that if a woman books with us we will look after her during her pregnancy and labour, and undertake her care, with her new baby, for 28 days afterwards.

We offer homebirth...

The House of Commons Select Committee produced a report, *Changing Childbirth*, on Maternity services in August 1993. In preparing the report, the committee listened to evidence from everyone involved – midwives, doctors, mothers and consumer organizations. The MPs evaluated the evidence, and came to the conclusion that hospital birth is not safer than homebirth for women having a normal pregnancy. We support this conclusion, and have worked with many women having homebirths.

We offer each client an individual service...

Independent midwives are flexible in their approach to clients, and try to fit the service to meet each woman's needs. We have some experience in the use of alternative therapies, and a lot of experience in active birth and alternative birthing positions, including waterbirths.

As professional practitioners, we are supervised by the Local Supervising Authority and the local Supervisors of Midwives. We carry our own equipment which has been approved by the local Supervisor, and our own drugs. We maintain a close professional relationship with our colleagues in the NHS, and we are trained to deal with any emergency which may arise until appropriate assistance can be obtained.

Your local independent midwife is:

APPENDIX II

Equipment List

Portable doppler fetal heart detector
Pinard stethoscope
Sphygmomanometer
Stethoscope
Urine testing sticks
Tape measure

Venepuncture equipment:
    tourniquet
    syringes and needles, or vacutainers
    blood bottles
    test request cards
    container to keep it all in
Plastic folders for notes

Sterile gloves
Thermometer
Inco pads
Entonox/oxygen equipment, including cylinder heads

Instruments, which should include:
    Spencer Wells or Kochers forceps x 2
    pair of large, sharp scissors
    pair of suture scissors
    stitch holder
    dissecting forceps
    speculum for high vaginal swabs
Sterilizable container with a well fitting lid

Syringes and needles
Sharps disposal container
Sterile mucous extractors – double chamber
Cotton wool packs, sterile and ordinary
Sterile gauze swabs, large and small

Urinary catheters (non-retaining)
Sanitary towels
Suture material
Sterile cord clamps
Amnihook

Drugs, including:
    Pethidine
    Syntometrine
    Ergometrine
    Lignocaine
    Local treatment for haemorrhoids
    Glycerine suppositories
    Sanispray hand cleanser, or a similar preparation

Transducer gel
Lubricant
Lotions
Baby scales
Umbilical cord tape
Lancets for Guthrie tests etc.
Cards for Guthrie Tests, serum bilirubin
Capillary tubes for serum bilirubin

A good camera
A heavy duty, bright torch

For emergencies, you'll need the following:
    Oxygen, maternal and neonatal
    Laryngoscope, with infant blade
    Laerdal bag and mask
    Airways – adult and neonatal
    IV catheter and giving set, with some sticky plaster
    IV fluid, e.g. Hartmann's and gelufusin

Bags to carry all this

APPENDIX III

Midwifery Notes

NAME _ _ _ _ _ _ _ _ _ _ _ _ _ _ DOB _ _ / _ _ / _ _

ADDRESS _

OCCUPATION _

PHONE _

PARTNER _

PHONE _ _ _ _ _ _ _ _ _ _ _ OCCUPATION _ _ _ _ _ _

GP _

SURGERY _ _ _ _ _ _ _ _ PHONE _ _ _ _ _ _ _ _ _ _

———————————————

LSA _ _ _ _ _ _ _ _ _ _ SUPERVISOR _ _ _ _ _ _ _

HOSPITAL/HOME _ _ _ _ LOCAL UNIT _ _ _ _ _ _ _ _

DATE OF BOOKING _ _ _ _ _ _ _ _ _ _ _ _ _ _ _ _ _ _

———————————————

METHOD OF PAYMENT _ _ _ _ _ _ _ _ _ _ _ _ _ _ _ _ _

SIGNED (MIDWIFE) _ _ _ _ _ _ _ _ _ _ _ _ _ _ _ _ _ _

SIGNED (CLIENT) _ _ _ _ _ _ _ _ _ _ _ _ _ _ _ _ _ _ _

ANTENATAL RECORD

Gravida: Parity:

Date of last period: Usual cycle:

Normal length?   Normal loss?

Any subsequent bleeding?

EDD:

Blood group: Rhesus: Rubella:

Height: Booking weight:

Non-pregnant weight:

Dental care?

Smoker?   How much?   Alcohol?

Diet:

Exercise:

Previous pregnancies:

where born	gestation	mode	sex	weight	comment

Blood results

	Hb	Antibodies	AFP	TPHA	Other
Booking 28 weeks 36 weeks					

MEDICAL HISTORY

	client	partner
Hypertension		
Thromboembolism		
Heart disease		
Renal disease		
Cystitis		
Genital herpes		
Thrush		
Sexually transmitted diseases		
Diabetes		
Respiratory disorder		
Tuberculosis		
Epilepsy		
Migraine		
Psychiatric disorder		
Jaundice/hepatitis		

	client	partner
Rubella		
Thyroid		
Any allergies?		

Operations

Blood transfusion y/n   date   where

Any family medical problems?

Any problems this pregnancy?

Breastfeeding?

Nipples checked?

THIS PREGNANCY

DATE	GEST	FUNDUS	PRES/POS	F/H	BP	OED	URINE

Comment

LABOUR RECORD

Date/time called: Time arrived:

History:

Temperature: Pulse: B/P:

Initial examination:

Abdominal:

Vaginal:

Plan of action:

LABOUR PROGRESS

LABOUR SUMMARY
Type of delivery:

Presentation at delivery:

Membranes ruptured spontaneously/artificially:

               start   finish   total

1st stage:

2nd stage:

3rd stage:
                        TOTAL

Drugs given   Date/time

Placenta and membranes
Complete/incomplete/doubtful

No. of vessels in cord

Cord blood taken

TOTAL BLOOD LOSS

Perineum
Intact/tear/episiotomy

Sutured/not sutured

Post delivery observations
Temperature   Pulse   B/P   Fundus

Lochia   Passed urine

BABY

Date and time of birth

Sex   weight   head circumference

Resuscitation required

APGARS (some modification)

	0	1	2	1 min	5 min
Heart rate	absent	< 100	< 100		
Respirations	absent	slow/weak	lusty cry		
Muscle tone	limp	some tone	strong		
Reflexes	no response	withdraws	vigourous		
Colour	pale/blue	blue/pink	pink		
TOTALS					

Any abnormalities noted

POST DELIVERY OBSERVATIONS

Temperature: Colour:

Bowels open: Passes urine:

Feeding:

GP notified of birth:

POSTNATAL RECORD – BABY
Entries from mother and midwife

POSTNATAL RECORD – MOTHER
Entries from mother and midwife

APPENDIX IV

Letter to Supervisors

Mary Jones, RGN RM
Independent Midwife
27 Poplar Rise, Anychester

Ms Lobelia Graffham
Supervisor of Midwives
Anychester Hospital
Anychester

20/2/97

Dear Ms Graffham

This is to inform you that we have booked the following client for home delivery.

NAME: Kitty Breakwater

ADDRESS: 12, The Centile, Anychester

EDD   14/7/97

Gravida: 3   Para: 1

GP: Dr H Spindrift   Address: The Surgery, Muesli Close.

We shall, of course, keep you informed of her progress.

Yours sincerely

MARY JONES

A Proposal for the Establishment of a Maternity Centre

Introduction

We believe that there is a need for community maternity 'homes' which provide facilities for normal deliveries and/or postnatal care in response to the recent Parliamentary Select Committee report (Winterton Report, 1992).

We therefore propose that there be one pilot centre in an appropriately chosen demographic area, probably in an urban setting, close to the local NHS unit (close means within twenty minutes travelling time). This centre would be managed and run by two local independent midwives, and would be staffed by a small core group of midwives. They would be responsible for their own cases, and could also take the day-to-day responsibility for postnatal care of other clients residing at the centre.

Facilities should include:
- Consulting rooms
- Teaching room, and a seminar room
- A labour area, with a pool
- 4–6 postnatal rooms
- Scanning facilities (a small real-time scanner).

These facilities would be available to local midwives, whether independent or NHS, to care for women who want this service. We could consider renting space to alternative therapists and exercise teachers, which will increase our client pool. GPs would be encouraged to use the centre freely, as a base to do antenatal sessions, an opportunity to practise non-interventionist intrapartum care and as a lying-in facility for their clients. GPs will, of necessity, have to practise under the aegis of the NHS as we cannot insure them. We will establish sound professional relationships with our obstetrician colleagues, based on a mutual respect for our differing but complementary skills.

Contacts with local organizations will be of great importance such as the NCT, AIMS, Genscan (a GP 'club'), local women's groups, local RCM branches, GP surgeries, alternative practitioner associations, and so forth.

The care concept remains central to the plan – continuity of care, with high calibre midwives; good quality accommodation with all the necessary accoutrements such as constant access to quality food, and a service attitude from staff; a continuing commitment to education, by teaching through apprenticeships, study days, seminars and workshops; the essential skills and arts necessary to the safe, but minimally interventionist, practice of maternity care. We shall apply to the local schools of midwifery to offer our facilities and experience to midwives in training. Midwives wishing to avail themselves of the opportunity to practice to the full extent of their role would work from the centre under the mentorship of more experienced practitioners.

As soon as possible after opening the centre, a swimming pool, if there is not one on-site already, should be considered, even if only a hydrotherapy size pool can be afforded. This would be a major means of introducing the centre to potential users, and was the factor reported as the one that most women would use as an ancillary facility in a BMRB survey. It may well be possible to fund this through a grant from one of the medical charities, or the Department of Health.

A small creche is another ancillary facility that we would hope to have in place from the outset, which will be available to clients and to staff. In this way we hope to encourage diverse working practices such as jobshare, and part time work without loss of status. We would wish to offer evening antenatal appointments for the benefit of working women, and also evening parentcraft classes for couples.

We have to encourage women to take up as much of the service as meets their personal needs. By doing this they will feel that the centres are tailored and flexible, and we get the opportunity to begin to build a practice database upon which we would be able to base research, and conduct audits of care.

Each woman will have her own midwife, with a co-midwife as back up. The responsible midwife may be the woman's own community midwife, or a midwife working in the centre. The woman will have freedom to choose whichever midwife she wishes, so long as that midwife is in agreement. Whenever births take place in the centre, there will always be a second midwife in the centre in case help is needed.

In addition to the midwifery carried out at the centre, we would envisage the centre as a base for a specialist homebirth team (see Appendix 6) whose statistics and findings would be incorporated into the database at the centre. This would provide the team with a place to call home for messages, meetings, classes and storage, and would also enable them to avail themselves of professional support when they needed it.

Comments from obstetricians

Consultants spoken to in this area have been working on a review of local services which appears to be very close to the ideas contained in the Health Committee Report.

Comments from midwives

Midwives who currently practice in hospital could be divided into three groups.

1.   Those who were apprehensive at the idea of leaving the institutional confines were disbelieving of the research findings about safety, and tried to dismiss those findings on somewhat tenuous grounds. When challenged, several admitted that their anxieties lay in their lack of confidence in their own abilities to practise without a constant medical presence. It is probably not reasonable to expect this group of midwives to be able to adapt their practice to cope with the increased expectations raised by the report of the Health Committee, and they may well form the core of staff who continue to provide a hospital service.

2.   This group was made up of midwives who would welcome the opportunity to extend their role into the community, but who felt that they would need/prefer to initially practice under the aegis of a midwife who was confident in her own extended role. There were quite a few newly qualified midwives in this group.

3.   This group comprised those midwives, many of them mothers themselves, who greeted the concept of community centres with delight and enthusiasm. These are midwives who have been waiting for community posts to come up (a somewhat rare event); those who perceived opportunities to operate diverse working practices, whilst retaining their status (sadly, part-timers are often not as highly graded, nor do they have a place on the promotional scale like their full-time colleagues); and those relatively newly qualified midwives who are disheartened by the long haul in front of them before they can get out into the community. The last group were very enthusiastic

about the concept of 'apprenticing' themselves to more experienced midwives.

Community midwives were also mixed in their response. A few were concerned that they would now be expected to give intrapartum care which they did not wish to do, and a few who see work in the community as basically 'a nine to five job, which gives me the freedom to come and go in the day the way I want to'. Many others, however, gladly welcomed the concept as enhancing their own practice, giving women a really good alternative to hospital or home, and a chance to improve the general perceived quality of maternity care in the area. It has to be said that, with a few notable exceptions, most community midwives did not feel confident in their abilities to help mothers wanting a homebirth, and were reluctant to involve themselves in this area.

Eight midwives, not currently practising, were asked if they would use the centre in order to undertake an apprenticeship or to re-establish practice. Seven said that they would give it serious consideration, and all eight said that they would consider it if there were a creche.

Comments from GPs

Four surgeries who have a reputation for being pro-choice in Southampton were asked for responses. Three of the four were very positive. One commented that he felt his practice would be extremely interested if the centres were non profit making, another decided that he would like to go on a workshop to learn how to put on forceps in anticipation of the centre opening! The third felt that it would answer a great many of his misgivings over the currently available system. The fourth explained that at his practice they did no intrapartum work, as they considered that they didn't get enough practice to be reliable. They appeared rather interested in the idea of practical training under the support and guidance of experienced midwives. All of them felt, as an initial response, that they would feel able to advise their clients of the option of care/delivery at the centre.

A number of low risk women could be allocated to the centre midwives, plus a certain percentage booked by those community midwives who would like to offer this service to their clients. Exact numbers to be agreed later, but a working hypothesis might begin at about five deliveries a week, working up to two deliveries per week per midwife when established.

We propose, therefore, that the DHA as a matter of urgency, consider the establishment of a community maternity centre along the lines of that recommended by the Health Committee.

APPENDIX VI

A Proposal for the Establishment of a Homebirth Service

We propose that, in the light of the recent Health Committee report (*Changing Childbirth*, 1993), the health authority examine its contracts for homebirths in the area.

Currently, only a very small percentage (less than one per cent) of all births occur at home. This figure includes unplanned homebirths for whom the Perinatal Mortality Rate (PMR) is statistically higher than that for planned homebirths. The evidence in the NPEU booklet 'Where to be born' (NPEU, 1987) suggests that for planned homebirth with low risk mothers, the PMR and morbidity rates are substantially lower than for the same group of women in a hospital setting. In Holland, 35 per cent of all births are at home, with a PMR that supports the contention that planned homebirth is a wholly safe option. We also have evidence that there are about 10–11 per cent of women who would have liked to deliver at home, but who felt pressurized by various means into abandoning their plans.

If we are to accept that homebirth is a safe birthing option for healthy women having healthy pregnancies, we must make proper provision for those women to be delivered by competent and confident attendants. It is important to note that although all midwives have theoretical responsibility to attend homebirths, in practice, very few do. The idea of homebirth is hedged around by the fears that professionals have, which they tend to impose on women who request to deliver at home. This baseless fear has lead many women who might have been happy and content giving birth at home, to feel as if they are victims of the system, forced into hospital.

As independent midwives, we do not share these fears about homebirth. This is a known and familiar working setting for us, and we actively encourage women to give birth where they feel happiest and most secure. With the above statistics in mind, we would like to propose a radical new idea to the Health Authority. We would like to suggest that the Health Authority and local trusts consider using their independent midwives as founders of a specialist homebirth team, with responsibility for those women wishing to have home deliveries in the area and for whom there is no midwife experienced in homebirth available. We would offer the following as a basis for discussion:

Practice

Independent midwives would retain their independent status, and their autonomous practice. They would be self-employed, and their practice would be overseen by the local Supervisors of Midwives as usual. The area covered would be that covered by the DHA, including all satellite clinics. A team of three midwives should be sufficient to cover the area initially, as a pilot scheme, which we anticipate would be for a period of at least a year. We would anticipate that clients would be accepted on a basis of one delivery/week/midwife. This could rise to a team of four when the concept is established.

Care

Independent midwives would offer total care to those women booked by them. This would include access to pathology departments for blood tests etc., and to the obstetric ultrasound department when required. Direct right of referral to obstetricians would be essential, as it is assumed that not all women booked for homebirth would have GP cover. The new Health Committee Report talks of the importance of encouraging midwives to practice to the full extent of their role, and this includes the duty they have to practise on their own responsibility.

It is also assumed that some women will be self-referring, and it would be necessary for the homebirth team to have a right of veto over clients they felt were unsuitable for home delivery. That said, it would be a feature of the care offered by the team that they would be able to offer hospital delivery (with concomitant continuity of care) for those women assessed as unsuitable for home delivery. We would also recommend that no woman should be refused a homebirth before being assessed by the homebirth midwives.

Education

All midwives are responsible for keeping themselves up to date with developments in practice, and for attending statutory refresher days/courses. It is of supreme importance that we can demonstrate our practice to be research-based and this is a duty which we welcome.

We would expect to have student midwives allocated to us in as supernumary a position as seems appropriate to the approved midwife tutor. We would also welcome the chance to offer preceptorship and experience to newly qualified midwives which would bolster their confidence in homebirths as well as augmenting their professional experience.

Finance

We would suggest that the midwives be funded in a similar way to GPs. The establishment of the team would be funded by the DHA with the exception of equipment. Each midwife will supply, and be responsible for, the acquisition and maintenance of her own equipment. There are a number of charitable sources who have expressed an interest in the idea that we are proposing, and it is suggested that an application be made to bodies such as the Kings Fund or the Department of Health for financial assistance with the running costs of the team, for the duration of the pilot period. We would suggest two years as a period which would enable an accurate assessment of the scheme's viability. In this length of time, the midwives would be able to establish a database, and engage in practice audits which would be of immense value to midwifery research.

The midwives would be paid an agreed fee on a per client basis. They would also require a working budget for drugs, consumables, blood tests, scans etc. They would need efficient transport, and so we recommend that they be admitted to the DHA's lease car package. It is also expected that the DHA would fund the cost of statutory professional refresher courses.

It is important to note that it is notoriously difficult, if not impossible, under the current system to estimate accurately the cost to the health authority of each maternity client. With a significant increase in the numbers of homebirths, we must, instead of looking at a comparison of costs, look at the savings which can be made under this new regime.

Savings can be made in the following areas:

1. Costs of pain relief are less in homebirths.
2. There are fewer hospital admissions in this group of clients, and there are no postnatal hospital expenses.
3. Less obstetric intervention, fewer consultation costs.
4. Costs of drugs are less (e.g. syntocinon, antibiotics).
5. Equipment/consumables costs are less.
6. Indemnity insurance costs are born by the individual midwives (£2.5m).
7. If transfer is necessary, midwifery costs are saved by having the independent midwife continue to provide care.

APPENDIX VII

Useful Contact Addresses

Association for Improvements in Maternity Services
40 Kingswood Avenue
London
NW6 6LS
0181 960 5585

Association of Radical Midwives
62 Greetby Hill
Ormskirk
Lancs
L39 2DT
01695 572776

English National Board
Victory House
Tottenham Court Road
London
W1P 0HA
0171 388 3131

Independent Midwives Association
94 Auckland Road
Upper Norwood
London
SE19 2DB
0181 406 3172

Maternity Alliance
45 Beech Street
London
E2CP 2LX
0171 837 1265

MIDIRS
9 Elmdale Road
Clifton
Bristol
BS8 1BR
01179 251791

National Board of Scotland
22 Queen's Street
Edinburgh
EH2 1JX
0131 226 7371

National Childbirth Trust
Alexandra House
Oldham Terrace
Acton
London
W3 6NH
0181 992 8637

Northern Ireland National Board
RAC House
79 Chester Street
Belfast
BT1 4JE
01232 238152

Royal College of Midwives
15 Mansfield Street
London W1
0171 872 5100

Society to Support Home Confinements
Lydgate
Lydgate Lane
Wolsingham
Durham
01388 528044

UKCC
23 Portland Place
London
W1N 3AF
0171 637 7181

Welsh National Board
Floor 13
Pearl Assurance
Greyfriars Road
Cardiff
CF1 3RT
01222 395535

Index

The Independent Midwife

A GUIDE TO INDEPENDENT MIDWIFERY PRACTICE

Lesley Hobbs

BA (Hons), SRN, RMN, RM

Books for Midwives Press

An imprint of Hodder and Stoughton Ltd.

**For Gregory, Georgia and Susannah, whose fault it
was that I started in midwifery in the first place**

*Published by Books for Midwives Press, 174a Ashley Road, Hale, Cheshire,
WA15 9SF, England*

© Hobbs, 1997

Second edition

ISBN 1-898507-59-7

British Library Cataloguing in Publication Data
A catalogue record for this book is available from the British Library

Printed by Interprint Limited, Malta